Dedicated to Angela, Madison, Caitlin, and Hannah for their love and support, and to God for the opportunity and ability.

—Phil Page

To Gail for her continued love and support.

—Todd Ellenbecker

Contents.............................

Exercise Finder   vii

Preface   xiii

Acknowledgments   xv

1   Strength Training With Elastic Resistance   1

2   Shoulders and Arms   12

3   Chest and Upper Back   34

4   Abdominals and Lower Back   56

5   Hips and Thighs   80

Strength Band Training

Phil Page, MS, PT, ATC, CSCS
Todd Ellenbecker, MS, PT, SCS, OCS, CSCS

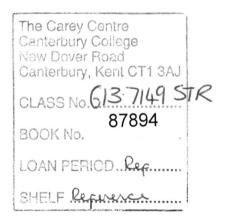

Canterbury College

87894

Library of Congress Cataloging-in-Publication Data

Page, Phil, 1967-
  Strength band training / Phil Page and Todd Ellenbecker.
    p. cm.
  Includes bibliographical references.
  ISBN 0-7360-5493-6 (soft cover)
  1. Isometric exercise. 2. Rubber bands. I. Ellenbecker, Todd, 1962- Title.
  RA781.2.P34 2005
  613.7'149--dc22

2004010169

ISBN: 0-7360-5493-6

Acquisitions Editor: Martin Barnard; **Managing Editor:** Wendy McLaughlin; **Assistant Editor:** Kim Thoren; **Copyeditor:** Nancy Wallace Humes; **Proofreader:** Pam Johnson; **Permission Manager:** Toni Harte; **Graphic Designer:** Nancy Rasmus; **Cover Designer:** Keith Blomberg; **Photographer (cover):** © The Hygenic Corporation; **Photographer (interior):** Kelly Huff, except for the following: page 4 © Kristiane Vey/jump; page 56 © Denis Light/Light Photographic; page 80 © Bruce Coleman; page 122 © Human Kinetics; page 151 © Joe McDonald/Bruce Coleman, Inc.; **Art Manager:** Kareema McLendon; **Printer:** Versa Press

Human Kinetics books are available at special discounts for bulk purchase. Special editions or book excerpts can also be created to specification. For details, contact the Special Sales Manager at Human Kinetics.

Printed in the United States of America   10 9 8 7 6 5 4 3 2

Human Kinetics
Web site: www.HumanKinetics.com

United States: Human Kinetics
P.O. Box 5076
Champaign, IL 61825-5076
800-747-4457
e-mail: humank@hkusa.com

Canada: Human Kinetics
475 Devonshire Road Unit 100
Windsor, ON N8Y 2L5
800-465-7301 (in Canada only)
e-mail: orders@hkcanada.com

Europe: Human Kinetics
107 Bradford Road
Stanningley
Leeds LS28 6AT, United Kingdom
+44 (0) 113 255 5665
e-mail: hk@hkeurope.com

Australia: Human Kinetics
57A Price Avenue
Lower Mitcham, South Australia 5062
08 8277 1555
e-mail: liaw@hkaustralia.com

New Zealand: Human Kinetics
Division of Sports Distributors NZ Ltd.
P.O. Box 300 226 Albany
North Shore City
Auckland
0064 9 448 1207
e-mail: info@humankinetics.co.nz

6   Lower Legs and Ankles   100

7   Combination and Circuit Training   110

8   Power, Agility, and Speed Exercises   120

9   Stretching Exercises   140

10   Functional Training Programs   150

11   Training on the Road   200

Bibliography   203

About the Authors   205

Exercise Finder.......................

Chapter 2   Page

Lateral raise	14
Front raise	16
Overhead press	18
Shoulder internal and external rotation	20
Diagonal flexion (PNF)	22
Diagonal extension (PNF)	24
Elbow curl	26
Elbow extension	28
Wrist flexion and extension	30
Supination and pronation	32

Chapter 3

Bench press	36
Seated row	38
Chest fly	40
Reverse fly	42
Lat pulldown	44
Shrug	46
Bent-over row	48
Chest pullover	50
Push-up	52
Dip	54

Chapter 4

Curl-up	58
Lower-abdominal crunch	60

Trunk twist   62

Back extension   64

Side bend   66

Side bridge   68

Bridge   70

Lift   72

Chop   74

Quadruped stabilization   76

Supine stabilization   78

Chapter 5

Hip flexion   82

Hip extension   84

Hip abduction   86

Hip internal and external rotation   88

Knee extension   90

Knee flexion   92

Leg press   94

Squat   96

Lunge   98

Chapter 6

Dorsiflexion   102

Plantar flexion   104

Inversion   106

Eversion   108

Chapter 8

Assisted throwing   125

Resisted forward running   126

Resisted backward running   127

Resisted lateral running   128

Resisted carioca   129

Resisted lateral movement   130

Resisted lateral jump step plyometric   131

External rotation plyometric 90/90 position   132

Squat with elastic band on barbell   133

Deadlift with elastic band on barbell   134

Arm acceleration drill (PNF D2 diagonal)   135

Step jump with elastic resistance   136

Assisted sprinting   137

Lateral bounding   138

Resisted step-up and step-over   139

Chapter 9

Upper trapezius   142

Pectoralis major   143

Quadriceps and rectus femoris   144

Iliotibial band   145

Hip flexors and iliopsoas   146

Piriformis   147

Hamstrings   148

Gastrocnemius and soleus   149

Chapter 10

Standing extension with retraction (Thumb out)   153

Linton external rotation   154

Batting simulation two-hand rotation   155

Lateral step with glove   156

Throwing simulation   157

Monster walk 159

Explosion out of three-point stance 160

Total-body extension 161

Rip 162

Closed-chain hip rotation 164

Abduction pattern with soccer ball 165

Basic kicking diagonal 166

Reciprocal arm and leg 167

Concentric and eccentric hamstrings 168

Throw-in simulation and overhead pass 169

Wrist radial deviation 171

Wrist ulnar deviation 172

Unilateral row with side bridge 173

Serratus punch 174

Open stance forehand resisted movement with racket 175

Elbow extension with shoulder abduction (Serve simulation) 176

Seated ball rotation with racket 177

Horizontal abduction (Backhand) 178

Golf-swing acceleration 180

Golf-swing take-back with resistance 181

Single-leg knee bend 183

Balance squat with chair 184

Tuck squat 185

Side to side lateral agility 186

Double-leg resisted squat 187

Biceps curl at 90 degrees shoulder flexion 189

Pull-through 190

Triceps extension (Swim position) 191

Squat walk 194

Skating stride   195

Resisted slide and stride   196

Resisted slap shot (Take-back position)   197

Resisted slap shot (Follow-through position)   198

Wrist shot (Start and end position)   199

Preface.............................

Strength training, or resistive exercise, has been recognized as an important part of any fitness or training program. In fact, the American College of Sports Medicine recommends strength training at least two days a week for both young and older adults. This practical, easy-to-use book is designed to help you develop a specific exercise program for your fitness or sports-training needs using a simple rubber band.

Elastic resistance training (ERT) has been used for nearly a century in fitness programs. For the past 25 years, it's been used mainly by rehabilitation professionals to help patients regain strength after an injury. Most recently, however, ERT has gained popularity in fitness, personal training, and sports-performance enhancement. Elastic resistance typically is achieved with either a large rubber band or a length of rubber tubing, and by its nature, it provides a variety of different exercises and applications. With a single piece of elastic resistance band or tubing, you can strengthen all the important muscle groups in the body and avoid the bulk and expense of resistance-exercise machines. For example, the same strengthening movement of a bench press can be performed using an elastic band. Another advantage is that there's no time wasted setting up equipment or moving to different machines. Because of its versatility, portability, and affordability, ERT is ideal for anyone involved in an exercise program. In addition, elastic resistance enhances any type of training you are interested in, from strengthening to flexibility to speed and agility. Best of all, you can put elastic bands in your pocket or gym bag and take them anywhere!

This book is your complete guide to working out with elastic bands and tubing in any fitness or sports program. The exercises are designed to strengthen every major muscle group, and they can be substituted for popular resistance-training equipment. This book will introduce exercises developed by European therapists and trainers focusing on improving balance and core strength within traditional exercises. New methods of wrapping and the self-stabilization of elastic bands help to promote whole-body strength and more functional movement. Each chapter contains "base" exercises, names the target muscle, and gives exercise instructions. Variations are then described for each base exercise. Next, a "core emphasis" progression is provided for each base exercise, which is typically performed with less resistance than the base exercise because of the increased demands on the body's core. Finally, each exercise has a training tip to ensure proper form and performance.

The remaining chapters include a discussion on ERT in combination with other types of exercises such as circuit training and aquatic exercise, as well as applications for power, agility, and speed. We also give an explanation of how to use ERT for stretching, followed by programs for sport-specific applications such as baseball, football, and soccer and workouts for the traveler. With elastic resistance, you are limited only by your imagination in what you can do!

Acknowledgments....................

We would like to thank the Hygenic Corporation for its continued support of research and education.

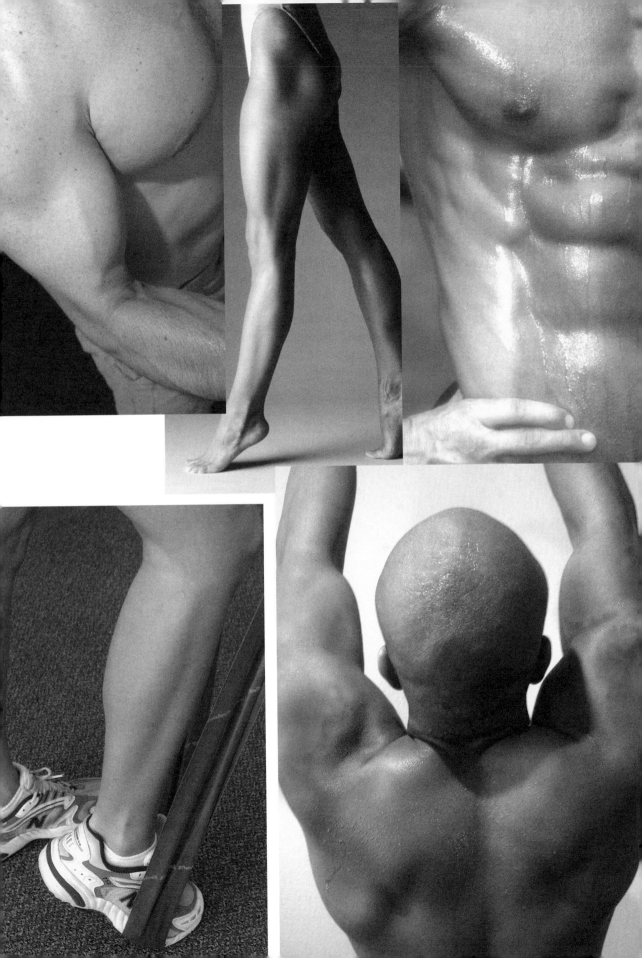

Chapter 1...............................

Strength Training With Elastic Resistance

The secret to elastic resistance exercise is a simple one. As the elastic band is stretched, the resistance increases. This resistance provides a progressive stimulus to the muscle to build strength and help increase muscle mass. Elastic resistance training (ERT) can work single or multiple joints at one time, making exercises more functional and efficient. With regular exercise machines and dumbbells, gravity (isotonic resistance) is the force opposing the weights, and often the user is limited to one particular exercise per machine. Elastic resistance, on the other hand, doesn't rely on gravity; rather, its resistance depends on how far the band or tubing is stretched (see table 1.1 and figure 1.1). And unlike on machines, many different exercises can be performed with a single band or tube, and the resistance is easily progressed by moving to the next level of difficulty, denoted by the color of band or tube. Figure 1.2 (page 3) shows that band resistance increases in the color progression of the Thera-Band brand by 20 to 30 percent as the bands are stretched to twice their resting length (100% elongation). One exercise band can be used to strengthen all the major muscle groups with exercises such as the bench press, seated row, upright row, lat pulldown, leg press, knee extension, and hamstring curl. Elastic bands can also help strengthen specific muscles that machines miss, such as the rotator cuff. In addition, bands can be used to perform flexibility and balance exercises, or to simulate sport-specific movements.

As recommended by the American College of Sports Medicine, strength training is an important part of any well-rounded exercise program. Research proves that ERT provides as much benefit in strength gains as those achieved on expensive and cumbersome weight-training equipment. Simply performing an exercise program for as few as six weeks with elastic resistance can increase strength by 10 to 30 percent. The added benefits of ERT include increased muscle mass, power, and endurance and decreased body fat. In fact, strength training of the legs with elastic resistance can even improve balance, gait, and mobility.

The chapters in this book provide functional activities and specific exercises to strengthen all major muscle groups. The target muscle is named for each exercise, followed by instructions and tips for proper movements. Be sure to

1

Table 1.1 Levels of Resistance for Thera-Band (in pounds of force)

Percent elonga-tion	Yellow	Red	Green	Blue	Black	Silver	Gold
25%	1	1.5	2	3	3.5	5	8
50%	2	2.5	3	4.5	6.	8.5	14
75%	2.5	3.5	4	6	8	11	18
100%	3	4	5	7	9.5	13	21.5
125%	3.5	4.5	5.5	8	11	15	24.5
150%	4	5	6.5	9	12.5	17	27.5
175%	4.5	5.5	7	10	13.5	19	30.5
200%	5	6	8	11	15	21	33.5
225%	5.5	6.5	9	12	16	23	36.5
250%	6	7	9.5	13.5	17.5	25.5	40

perform the movements properly before adding resistance. Most important, use a resistance that allows completion of the target repetitions without excessive fatigue and with proper form.

As with any resistance training modality, elastic resistance offers several advantages and disadvantages to be considered when developing a strengthening program. The greatest advantages of elastic resistance are its portability,

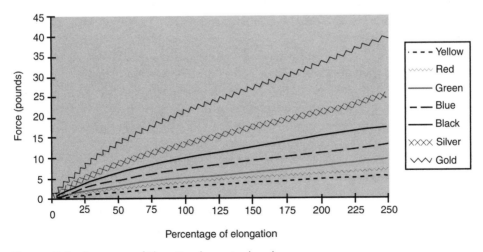

Figure 1.1 Resistance of Thera-Band exercise bands.

affordability, and versatility. Unlike isotonic resistance (free weights, machines, pulleys), elastic resistance relies on the tension within the band rather than the pull of gravity. While isotonic-resistance exercises are typically limited to upward movements (movements against gravity), elastic resistance offers many more movements and directions of motion for exercises (such as side to side). This imparts a higher level of neuromuscular control compared with specific machines. Elastic resistance exercises multiple joints and planes in the more functional standing position (rather than the sitting position on machines), which causes more core training than the same machine-based exercise. The "core" area includes the abdominal and low back area, as well as the hips. In addition, it's much harder to "cheat" with an elastic resistance exercise because momentum doesn't play a role, as it can when lifting weights. In contrast to pulley- and machine-based resistance, elastic resistance offers inherent and smoother eccentric (negative) resistance during the return-phase of the movement, thus stimulating the anti-gravity function of muscles; that is, the role of muscles in supporting body segments in an upright position against the pull of gravity. Finally, elastic bands also allow faster movements and plyometric exercises, while isotonic resistance and machines do not.

Some have said that training with bands doesn't work, stating that the increasing force of the bands is opposite to the increasing-decreasing bell-shaped muscular-strength curve. Their argument is that the band is at its greatest force when the muscle is least able to produce force at end range. However, clinical research has shown that the strength curve produced by elastic resistance is, in fact, similar to strength curves of human joints. In addition, elastic resistance exercises are not restricted by a single plane of motion, as typical isotonic exercises are. Elastic resistance offers multiple planes of resistance—the frontal, sagittal, and transverse planes—offering resistance to both isolated and integrated movements. Elastic resistance is uniquely suited

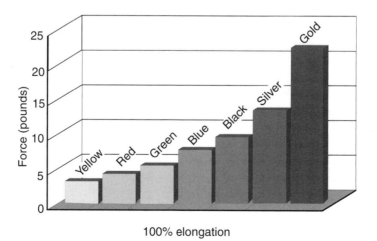

Figure 1.2   Force (in pounds) of Thera-Band elastic bands at 100% elongation.

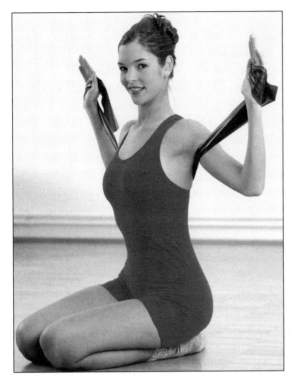

Elastic bands are versatile, allowing a variety of exercises.

for replicating whole-body, multiple-joint movements of functional activities such as simulated throwing, lifting, and running. Finally, several research studies have noted improvements in function and mobility in different age groups. Based on the biomechanical and clinical evidence, elastic resistance is definitely ideal for functional training.

Some disadvantages of the bands are durability. Unfortunately, elastic bands and tubing occasionally break. While they are more subject to wear and tear than isotonic weights, elastic resistance products have a longer clinical life because of advances in manufacturing. Care must be taken to inspect bands regularly and to avoid objects that can cause damage. Be sure the bands are securely attached so they don't snap back and cause injury. It's also difficult to quantify the specific resistance of an elastic band compared with an isotonic weight. For example, a particular band can't be equated to the specific weight of a dumbbell; the force produced by each band depends on how much it is stretched. Elastic bands are not toys, so children should use them only with supervision. It's safe to say, however, that the advantages far outweigh the disadvantages.

Bands Versus Tubing

Some have asked whether there's a difference between bands and tubing. In general, the same color bands and tubing from the same manufacturer tend to have the same resistance levels. Be aware, however, that resistance levels do vary among different manufacturers. Physiologically and biomechanically, there are no differences between bands and tubing in terms of resistance training stimulus. Most of the time, using bands or tubing is a matter of personal preference: Bands tend to be preferred for lower-body exercises and tubing for upper-extremity exercises.

A benefit of exercising with a band is that it can simply be wrapped around the hand or a part of the body rather than attached to an object (see figure 1.3a-b). Tubing sometimes has a tendency to "cut" into the skin when wrapped

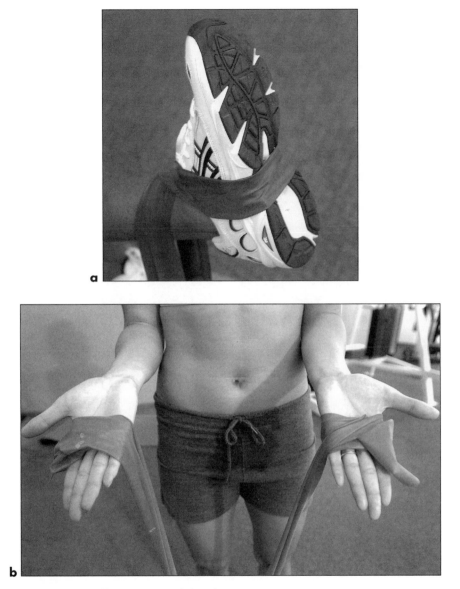

Figure 1.3   *(a)* Ankle wrappings, *(b)* hand wrappings.

around the hand and to roll over bony areas during movement. Although not essential, accessories and attachments for the bands and tubing (see figure 1.4a-e) can increase the number of possible exercises. Regardless of how the end of the band is attached, it must be fastened securely to prevent injury. In general, however, accessories, such as handles, door anchors, and extremity straps are recommended for tubing exercises to avoid hand discomfort. Elastic bands and tubing also are provided in closed "loops" at specific fixed lengths, which are useful in looping around extremities rather than grasping or using handles.

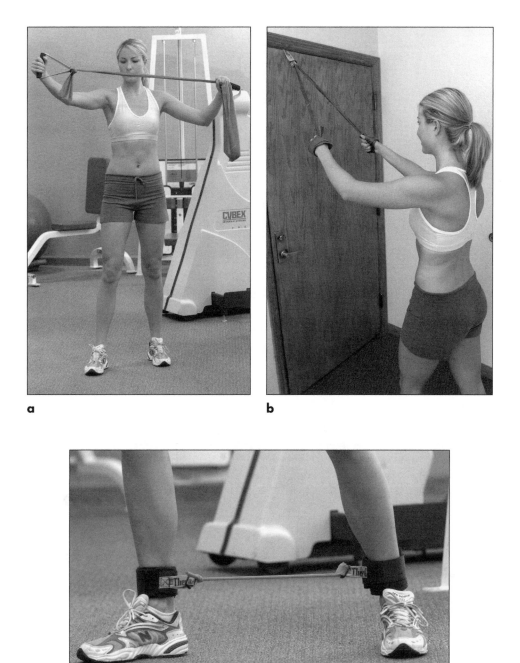

a

b

c

(continued)

Figure 1.4 Various accessories used in elastic resistance training: *(a)* handles, *(b)* door anchor, *(c)* extremity strap.

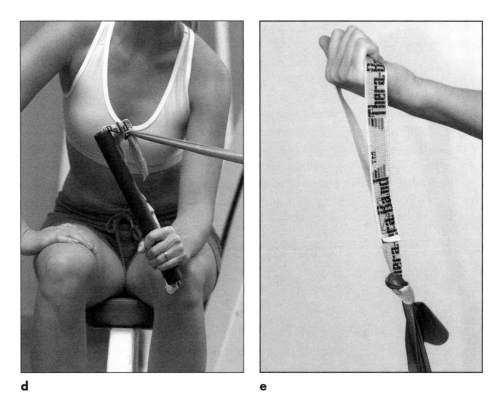

d   e

Figure 1.4 (continued)   Various accessories used in elastic resistance training: *(d)* sports handle, *(e)* assist strap.

Training Tips

ERT employs exercises as challenging as those performed on expensive gym equipment, and they can be done at home or while traveling. In fact, research has shown that elastic resistance exercises provide the same physiological benefits and outcomes as exercising with machines. In addition, ERT is free from the limitations of gravity, allowing performance of the same movements as those performed on a machine but isolating muscles in a totally different way, resulting in training more specific to the functional movement patterns.

By simply varying the level of resistance, the number of repetitions, and the pace of the exercise, a strengthening program can be tailored for weight loss, body toning, or general strength and conditioning, or to improve skills necessary for better sports performance. For example, using higher resistance with fewer repetitions will increase muscle size and strength, although using a lower resistance with more repetitions will help burn fat. Choose volume (sets and repetitions) and intensity (resistance level or color of band) to match workout goals. A dosing chart (see table 1.2) may be helpful in determining an exercise level. When using ERT, the "repetition maximum" (RM) method of determining exercise intensity is most useful. The RM is defined as the amount of resistance that can be moved a specific number of times to the point of fatigue. For example, a 1RM resistance is the amount of resistance that can be overcome only once, and a 10RM resistance would allow the user to move the resistance only 10 times. Traditional strength training programs typically use a %1RM method of prescribing exercise intensity (such as 60% 1RM), based on the amount of weight moved once, or a formula that predicts 1RM based on the number of repetitions completed at a specific resistance. By using a "multiple RM" method, the specific intensity of resistance can be quickly dosed individually with each exercise, without testing the 1RM or using a formula for each movement.

Table 1.2 Dosing Chart for Resistance Exercise

Goal	Intensity (% 1RM)	Intensity (Multiple RM)
Strength and power	85–90% 1 RM	3–6 RM
High-intensity endurance and speed	70–75% 1RM	10–12 RM
Low-intensity endurance	55–60% 1RM	20–25 RM

Start a program with lighter resistances to practice proper form and movements. Perform controlled, slow movements, and emphasize the "negative" (eccentric), or returning, part of the movement. Don't let the band snap back to the resting position. Improper movements often lead to joint injury and pain. Always balance the exercises for muscles on the front of the body with those for the back. For example, after a bench press, perform a seated row for the shoulder muscles. It's also essential to breathe properly during resistance exercises; don't hold your breath. As with any exercise program, proper warm-up and cool-down are recommended. Finally, proper posture is important for the full benefit of the exercises.

Precautions Before Beginning an Exercise Program . .

The following precautions should be observed.

- Get approval from a physician before starting resistance exercise.
- See a physical or occupational therapist beforehand if you have chronic musculoskeletal pain.
- Expect soreness at the beginning of any new exercise program.
- Contact your doctor if you have severe soreness for more than three days after a workout.

Safety First . . . .

It's important to consider safety when using any type of exercise equipment. Follow these guidelines when using bands and tubing.

- Inspect bands before each use, particularly at the attachment point, and replace if any show nicks or tears.
- Make sure band is securely fastened to the attachment point. For example, use a firmly closed door with the band pulling against its natural swing.
- Perform motions slowly and in control; don't let the band snap back.
- Avoid sharp objects, such as jewelry and fingernails, when using bands.
- Never point the band toward the face.
- Do not overstretch bands; never pull them more than three times their resting length. For example, a 2-foot band shouldn't stretch beyond 6 feet.
- Use latex-free bands for those with latex allergy.
- Keep your bands out of direct sunlight and heat, and avoid extremes of temperature.
- Wash your bands with a gentle soap and water.
- Lay bands flat to dry.
- Use handles (available separately) if you have trouble gripping the bands.

The Importance of Posture

It's important to maintain good overall body posture before, during, and after each movement. Emphasize proper spinal posture, because even when performing only shoulder exercises, good posture of the lower back and hips is essential to maintain a stable base for the shoulder muscles to work. Most of the exercises in this book are performed in a standing position to involve the core stabilizers more and to improve balance, but different postures can be used within the same movement for a different effect. For example, performing a bench press flat on a bench will use fewer core muscles than performing the same exercise on an exercise ball. The "athletic" standing posture (see figure 1.5) suggested in this book involves lumbar and cervical spines (lower back and neck) in neutral position; shoulders back and down; abdominals slightly contracted; navel pulled inward; knees soft, not locked; wrists in neutral position. An athletic posture promotes overall body stability and in this way improves activation of the core of the abdominals and lower back.

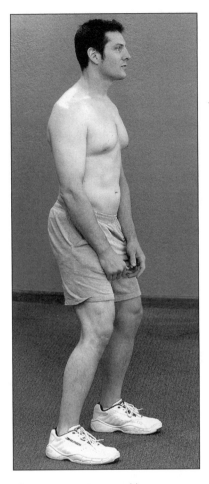

Figure 1.5   Proper athletic posture.

Quality Versus Quantity

Because these exercises put a demand on the whole body as well as on the joint they isolate, the body may be more prone to fatigue and tend to compensate with other muscles. With this in mind, exercises should be performed for "quality," not "quantity." It's crucial to remember that strength training is based not only on building muscle, but also on building the motor program (nervous system messages) for correct movements; therefore, proper posture and form is much more important than overall volume of training.

While overall posture is key, it's important to remember that the position of the band in relation to the person exercising will significantly affect the exercise. In particular, the stationary attachment point of the band (where the band is stretched from) and the subsequent line of pull, or "vector," of resistance will affect the overall strength curve as well as the stabilization requirements of the exercise. In general, the resistance band should be in the same plane of movement and parallel to the muscle fibers used in the movement. When performing a biceps curl, for example, the exercise band should be within the sagittal plane, parallel to the fibers of the biceps (see figure 1.6a-b). For a more detailed explanation of the biomechanics and correct positioning with elastic resistance training, see *The Scientific and Clinical Application of Elastic Resistance*, published by Human Kinetics.

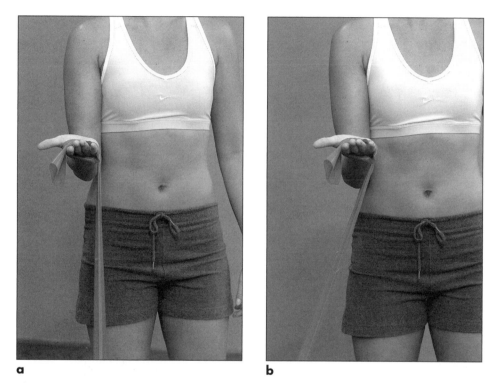

a   b

Figure 1.6   *(a)* Correct technique for the biceps exercise; *(b)* incorrect technique.

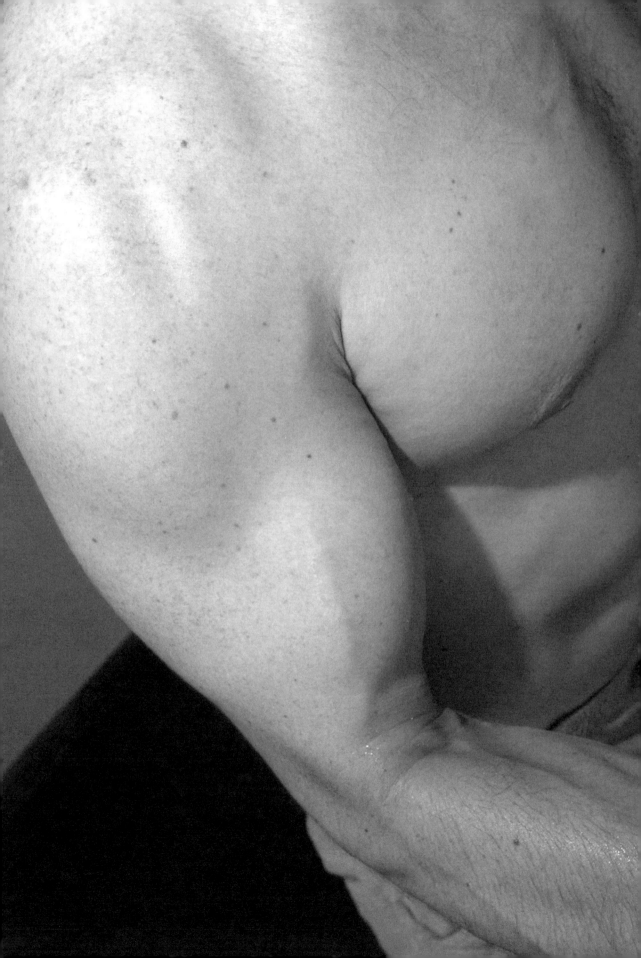

Chapter 2..............................
Shoulders and Arms

Traditionally, most elastic resistance training has been done on the shoulders. This is probably because it was easier to grasp rubber tubing and stretch it between the hands rather than attach it to the leg. Therefore, most applications and research of elastic resistance have been done on the upper extremities. Strengthening the shoulders and arms has functional implications during lifting, carrying, pushing, and reaching overhead. Strengthening the shoulders and arms may help prevent or rehabilitate shoulder injuries such as impingement, rotator cuff, tendinitis, tennis elbow, and carpal tunnel syndrome. In addition, sport-specific training of the shoulders and arms is important in throwing sports such as baseball and softball, in overhead sports such as tennis and volleyball, and in repetitive movement sports such as swimming. The unique properties of elastic resistance allow people to perform multiplanar (diagonal) movements, which are difficult to do with gravity-dependent machines. Remember to do the core emphasis exercises with slightly less resistance than you use in the basic exercises.

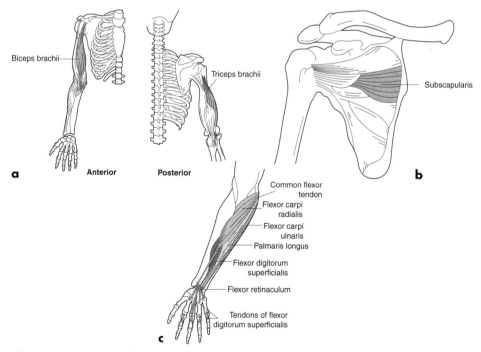

Figure 2.1 Muscles of the shoulders and arms. *(a)* shoulder joint muscles, *(b)* anterior view of shoulder, *(c)* wrist flexors.

LATERAL RAISE (Deltoids)

Stand on middle of long band. Wrap ends of band around hands. Bring bands around outside of feet, crossing bands between the knees. Lift bands overhead, keeping elbows straight *(a)*. Slowly return.

Variation

Empty-Can Raise (for rotator cuff): Bring arms forward slightly. Lift only to shoulder level, keeping thumbs pointed down and elbows straight.

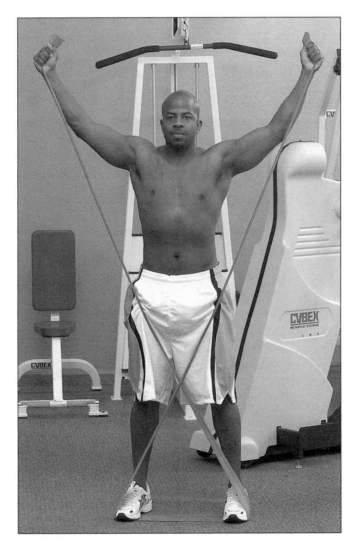

a

Core Emphasis

Forearm Wrap: Wrap band around forearm and perform lateral raise with elbow bent. Balance on leg that stabilizes band *(b)*. Stand on a foam surface for more challenge.

Training Tips

Keep shoulder blades down. Don't shrug shoulders during the movement. Keep abdominals tight and wrists straight.

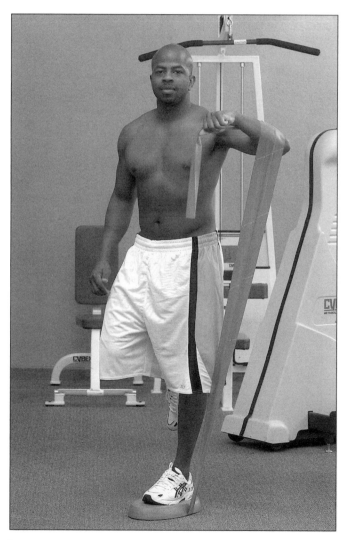

b

FRONT RAISE (Deltoids)

Stand on middle of long band. Wrap ends of band around hands. Bring bands forward and grasp at hips. Keep thumbs pointed upward. Lift bands overhead, keeping elbows straight *(a)*. Slowly return.

Variation

Staggered Step: Use a staggered step, with one foot in front of the other, and stabilize one end of band under forward foot. Pull bands overhead.

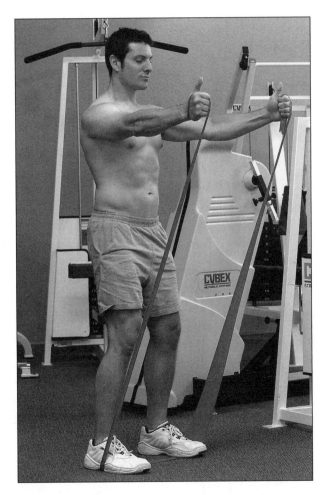

a

Core Emphasis

Forearm Wrap: Wrap band around forearm and perform a front raise with elbow bent. Simultaneously, lean forward while stabilizing back *(b)*.

Training Tips

Keep shoulder blades down. Don't shrug shoulders during the movement. Keep back straight and avoid arching backward. Keep abdominals tight and wrists straight. If you have a history of shoulder injury, limit the movement to 90 degrees, stopping at shoulder level.

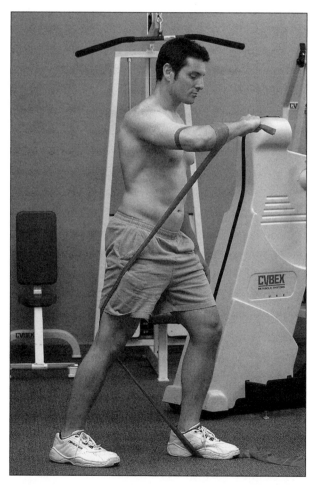

b

OVERHEAD PRESS (Deltoids, Upper Trapezius)

Stand on middle of long band. Wrap ends of band around hands. Lift bands overhead *(a)*. Slowly return.

Variation

Staggered Step: Use a staggered step, with one foot in front of the other, and stabilize one end of band under back foot. Pull bands overhead.

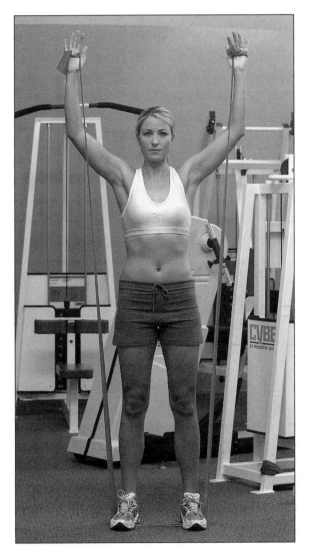

a

Core Emphasis

Stand on one leg to stabilize end of band. Pull band upward overhead, keeping back straight. Stand on a foam surface for more challenge (b).

Training Tips

Don't shrug shoulders during the movement. Keep back straight and avoid arching backward. Keep abdominals tight. If you have a history of shoulder injury, limit the movement to 90 degrees, stopping at shoulder level.

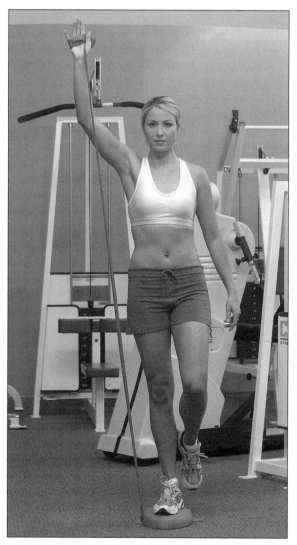

b

SHOULDER INTERNAL AND EXTERNAL ROTATION (Rotator Cuff)

Securely attach one end of band. Wrap other end around hand, with palm up. Keep elbow by the side and bent 90 degrees. Slowly pull band toward body and away from the attachment (a: external rotation; b:internal rotation). Slowly return.

Variation

90/90 Rotation: Lift arm so shoulder is at 90-degree angle to body; keep elbow at shoulder height. Pull band away from attachment, keeping shoulder and elbow bent 90 degrees (c).

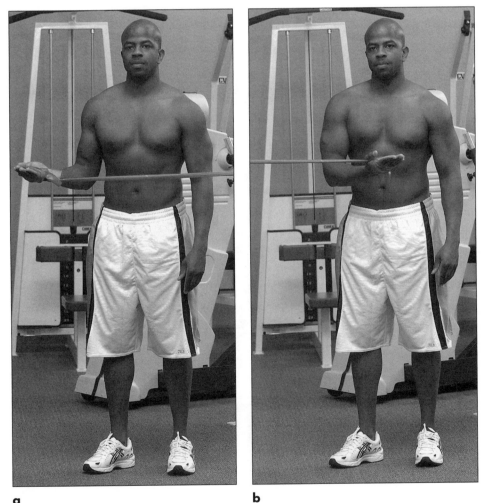

a   b

Core Emphasis

Stand on one leg while performing 90/90 rotation exercise. Stand on a foam surface for more challenge *(c)*.

Training Tips

Keep wrist straight and elbow bent at 90 degrees. Don't extend elbow or wrist to complete the motion. Keep trunk stationary. Don't rotate trunk to complete the motion.

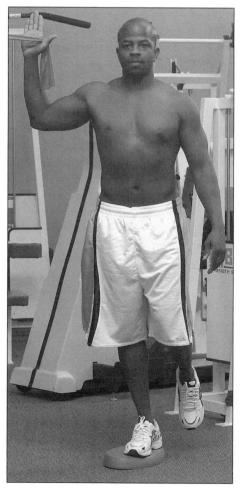

c

DIAGONAL FLEXION (PNF) (Deltoid, Rotator Cuff)

Securely attach one end of band. Wrap other end of band around hand. Pull band away from attachment, crossing body and keeping elbow straight (a). Slowly return.

Variation

Bilateral proprioceptive neuromuscular facilitation (PNF): Use two bands, and perform movement with both arms simultaneously (b).

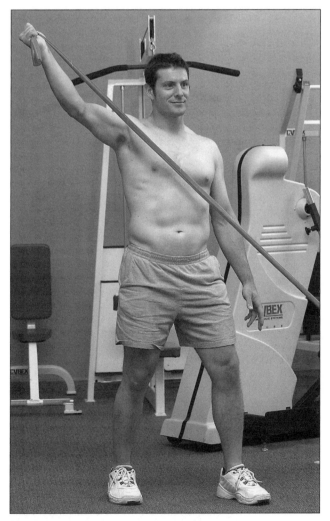

a

Core Emphasis

Stand on one leg to stabilize end of band while performing either the single-arm or bilateral PNF pattern exercise. Stand on a foam surface for more challenge *(b)*.

Training Tips

Keep back straight. Don't rotate trunk to complete motion. Keep abdominals tight.

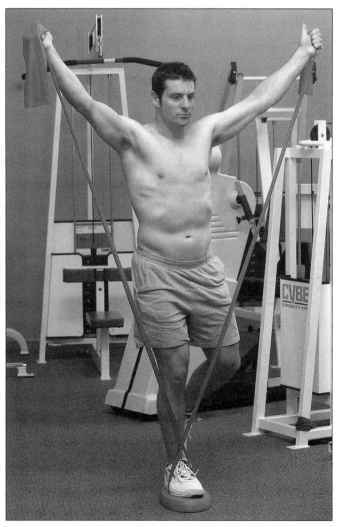

b

DIAGONAL EXTENSION (PNF)
(Anterior Shoulder)

Securely attach end of band. Wrap other end of band around hand. Pull band away from attachment, crossing body and keeping elbow straight *(a)*. Slowly return.

Variation

Bilateral PNF: Use two bands, and perform movement with both arms simultaneously.

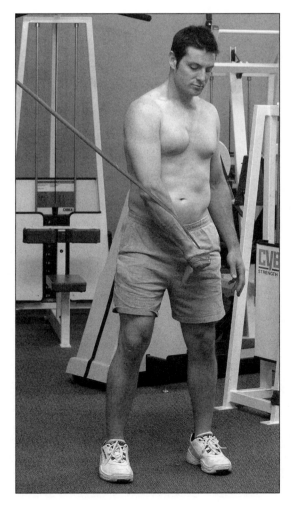

a

Core Emphasis

Stand on one leg to stabilize end of band while performing the single-arm or bilateral PNF pattern exercise. Stand on a foam surface for more challenge (b).

Training Tips

Keep back straight. Don't rotate trunk to complete motion. Keep abdominals tight.

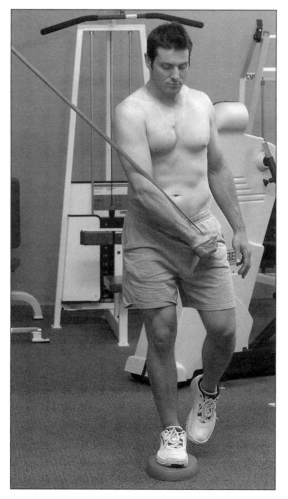

b

ELBOW CURL (Biceps)

Stand on middle of long band with one foot slightly in front of other. Wrap ends of band around hands. Keep palms up and elbows to sides. Bend elbows, lifting bands upward *(a)*. Slowly return.

Variation

90-Degree Concentration Curl: Securely attach one end of band at shoulder level. Lift shoulder forward to 90 degrees and grasp band with elbow straight. Keeping shoulder stable, bend elbow, bringing hand to shoulder *(b)*.

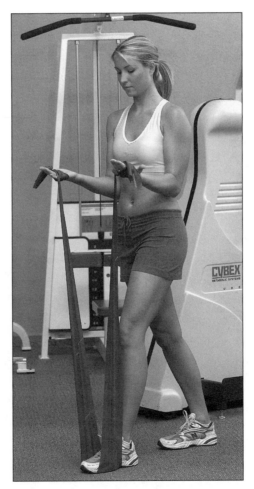

a

Core Emphasis

Stand on one leg while performing 90-degree concentration curl. Stand on a foam surface for more challenge *(b)*.

Training Tips

Keep shoulders and elbows steady, back straight, and don't lean backward. Keep abdominals tight and wrists straight. Don't bend wrists to complete motion.

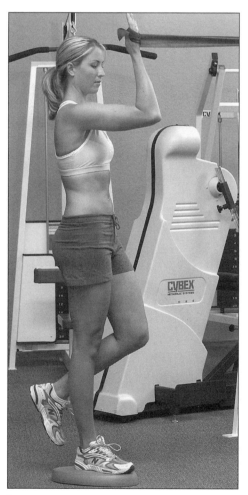

b

ELBOW EXTENSION (Triceps)

Securely attach middle of band in front and overhead. Wrap ends of band around hands. Begin with elbows bent at sides. Straighten elbows, keeping them at sides, palms facing backward *(a)*. Slowly return.

Variation

Overhead Press: Stand on one end of long band with back foot. Bring band up behind back, and grasp end overhead with shoulder elevated and elbow bent. Pull band upward, extending elbow.

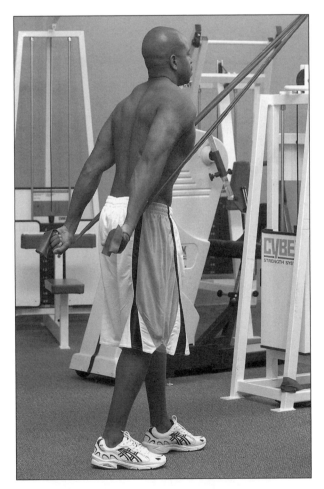

a

Core Emphasis

French Curl on Ball: Securely attach one end of band. Lie on exercise ball in tabletop position. Grasp band overhead, with your elbows at your sides. Extend elbow, keeping elbow and shoulder steady *(b)*.

Training Tips

Keep shoulders and elbows steady and back straight. Don't lean forward to complete the exercise. Keep abdominals tight and wrists straight.

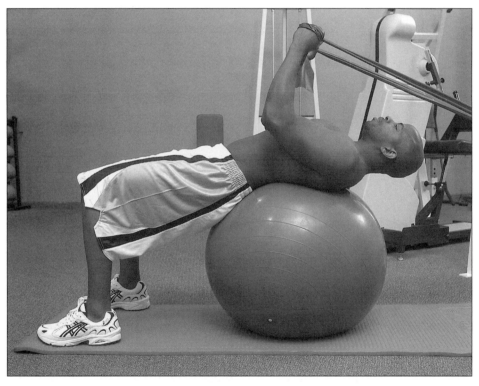

b

WRIST FLEXION AND EXTENSION
(Wrist Flexors and Extensors)

Attach both ends of band to a handle. Sit, and secure middle of band under feet. With elbow bent, stabilize forearm on thighs. Grasp handle with palm up for wrist flexion *(a)*, or palm down for wrist extension *(b)*. Bend wrist. Slowly return.

Variation

Grasp each end of band, hands about shoulder-width apart, palms facing each other. Extend both wrists at same time *(c)*. Slowly return.

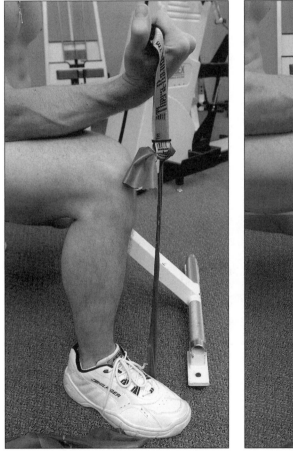

a

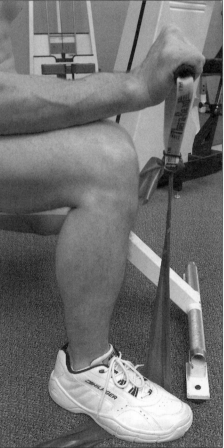

b

Core Emphasis

Stand on one leg while performing wrist extension exercise with both hands. Stand on a foam surface for more challenge *(c)*.

Training Tip

Keep elbows in one position during exercise. Don't use elbows to complete exercise.

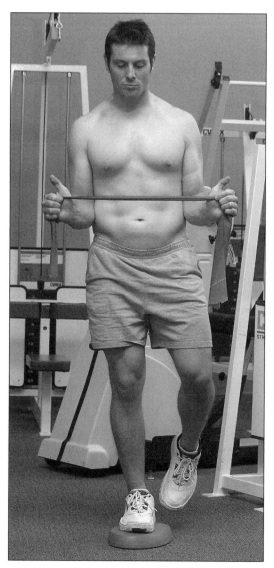

c

SUPINATION AND PRONATION
(Supinators and Pronators)

Securely attach one end of band. Attach other end to a handle. Grasp handle with thumb upward. Rotate forearms and turn palm up for supination (a), or palm down for pronation (b). Slowly return.

Variation

Grasp each end of band, hands about shoulder-width apart, palms facing each other. Rotate both forearms and turn palms upward at same time (c). Slowly return.

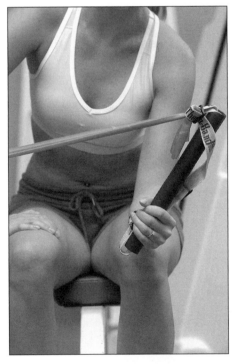

a

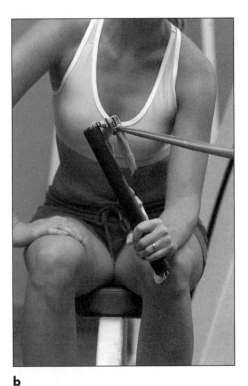

b

Core Emphasis

Stand on one leg while performing supination exercise with both hands. Stand on a foam surface for more challenge *(c)*.

Training Tip

Keep elbows in one position during exercise. Don't use elbows to complete the exercise.

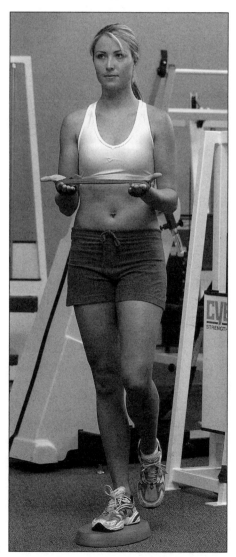

c

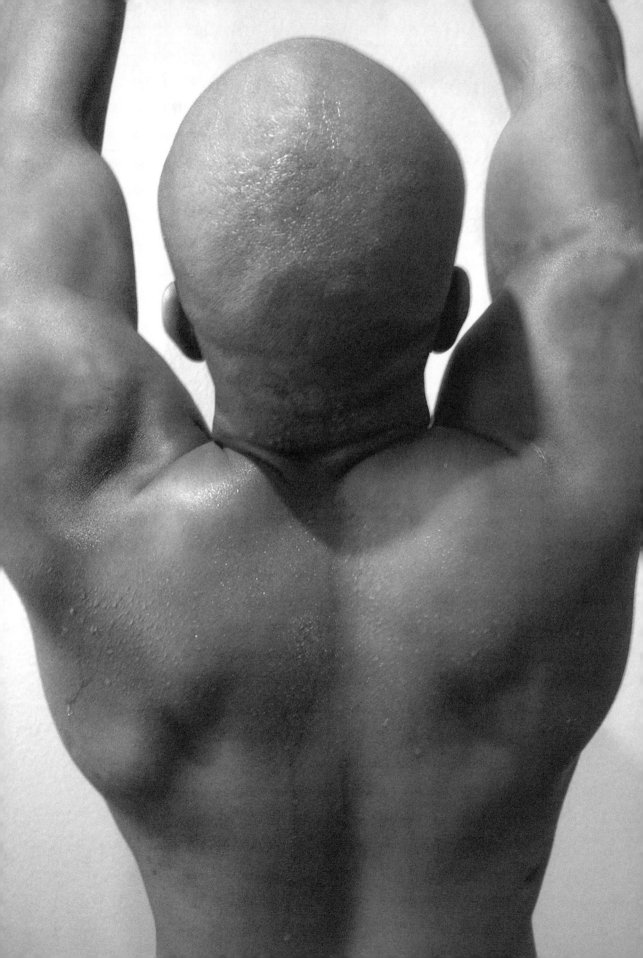

Chapter 3 . . . .

Chest and Upper Back

One of the most overworked areas of the body in strength training is the chest, mostly for aesthetic reasons. Unfortunately, few spend time to balance overworked chest muscles with the upper-back muscles. This imbalance can contribute to poor posture as well as shoulder and neck problems. Elastic resistance easily replicates the common exercises performed with traditional strengthening equipment, and these exercises are performed in a standing position, making workouts even more challenging. Strengthening the chest and upper back may help prevent or rehabilitate shoulder injuries as well as neck injuries. In addition, sport-specific training of the chest and upper back is important in overhead and throwing sports such as tennis and volleyball, baseball, and softball. Strengthening the chest and upper back has functional implications in carrying objects and in pushing or pulling movements. It's important to remember that the core emphasis exercises should be performed with slightly less resistance than the basic exercises.

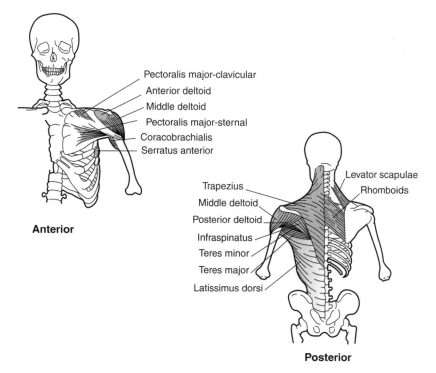

Anterior

- Pectoralis major-clavicular
- Anterior deltoid
- Middle deltoid
- Pectoralis major-sternal
- Coracobrachialis
- Serratus anterior

Posterior

- Trapezius
- Middle deltoid
- Posterior deltoid
- Infraspinatus
- Teres minor
- Teres major
- Latissimus dorsi
- Levator scapulae
- Rhomboids

Figure 3.1   Chest and upper back muscles.

BENCH PRESS (Pectoralis)

Secure middle of band to stationary object behind and at shoulder level. Face away from attachment. Use staggered step, with one leg slightly in front of the other. Grasp the handles at shoulder height with elbows bent. Extend arms, pushing bands forward *(a)*. Slowly return.

Variation

Change height of attachment of band for an incline press (lower attachment height) or decline press (higher attachment height).

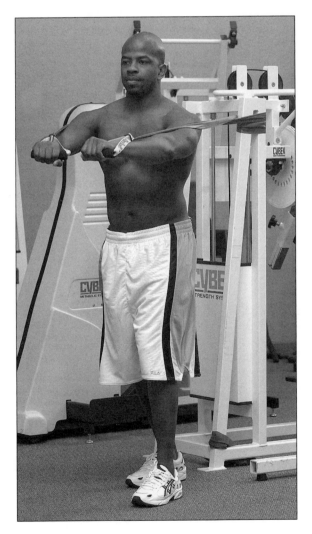

a

Core Emphasis

Stand on one leg while performing bench press exercise. Stand on a foam surface for more challenge *(b)*.

Training Tips

Keep shoulder blades down. Don't shrug shoulders during the movement. Keep back straight. Keep abdominals tight and wrists straight.

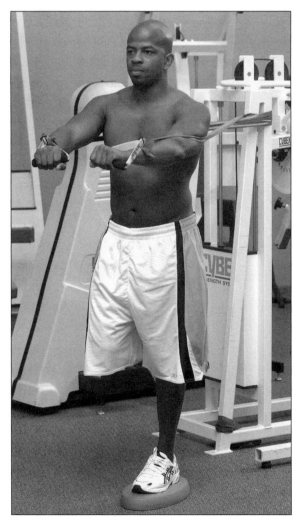

b

SEATED ROW (Rhomboids, Middle Trapezius)

Sit with legs extended. Wrap middle of band around outside of both feet, and cross bands. Grasp handles with elbows extended in front. Pull the band toward hips, bending elbows *(a)*. Slowly return.

Variation

Change height while pulling bands: hip level (low rows), lower-rib level (middle rows), and shoulder level (high rows).

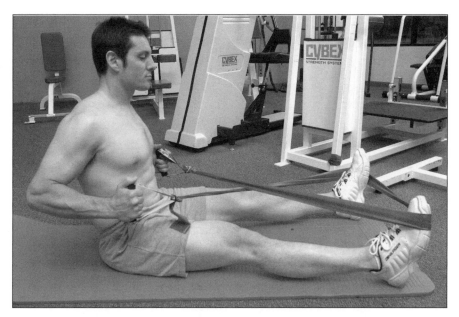

a

Core Emphasis

Secure middle of band to stationary object. Sit on exercise ball while performing seated row exercise *(b)*.

Training Tips

Keep back straight and abdominals tight. Keep wrists straight.

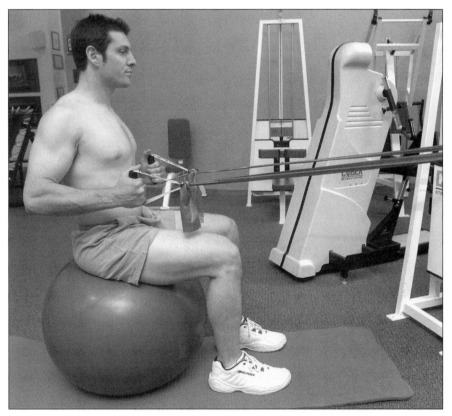

b

CHEST FLY (Pectoralis)

Secure middle of band to stationary object at shoulder level. Face away from attachment. Use staggered step, one leg slightly in front of other. Grasp the handles at shoulder height with elbows straight. Keep elbows straight and pull bands inward with palms facing each other (a). Slowly return.

Variation

Change height of attachment of band for an incline fly (lower attachment height) or decline fly (higher attachment height).

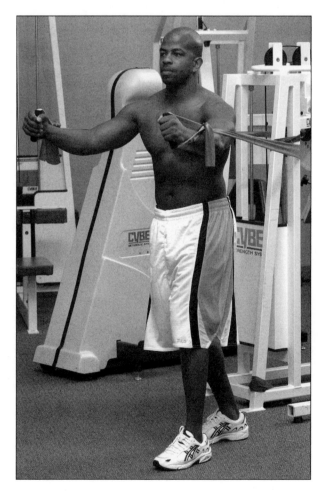

a

Core Emphasis

Stand on one leg while performing chest fly exercise. Stand on a foam surface for more challenge *(b)*.

Training Tips

Keep back straight and abdominals tight. Don't round shoulders. Keep wrists straight.

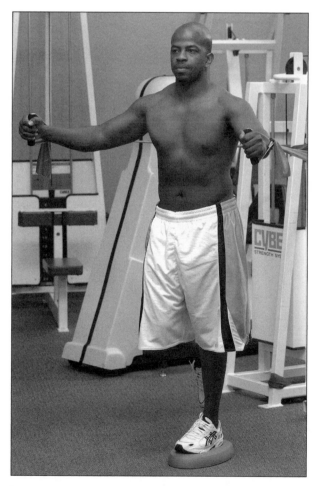

b

REVERSE FLY (Rhomboids, Middle Trapezius)

Secure middle of band to stationary object at shoulder level. Face attachment. Use staggered step, one leg slightly in front of other. Grasp the handles at shoulder height with elbows straight. Keep elbows straight and pull bands outward (a). Slowly return.

Variation

Change height of attachment of band for an incline fly (lower attachment height) or decline fly (higher attachment height).

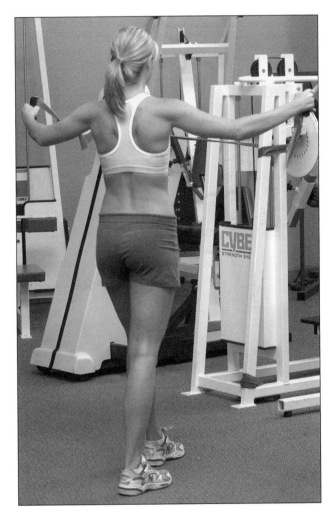

a

Core Emphasis

Stand on one leg while performing reverse fly exercise. Stand on a foam surface for more challenge *(b)*.

Training Tips

Keep back straight and abdominals tight. Don't round shoulders. Keep wrists straight.

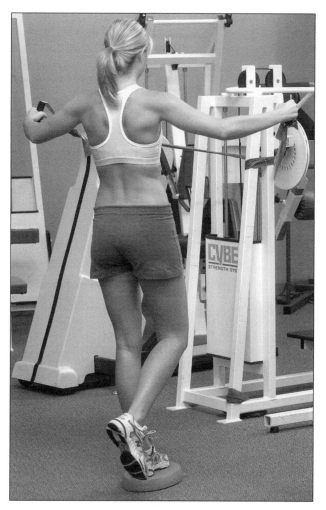

b

LAT PULLDOWN (Latissimus Dorsi)

Secure middle of band to stationary object above shoulder level. Face attachment. Use staggered step, one leg slightly in front of other. Grasp the handles above shoulder height with arms extended in front. Bend elbows and bring hands to chest, pulling the bands down and back *(a)*. Slowly return.

Variation

Begin with elbows straight above shoulder level. Keep elbows straight while extending arms downward.

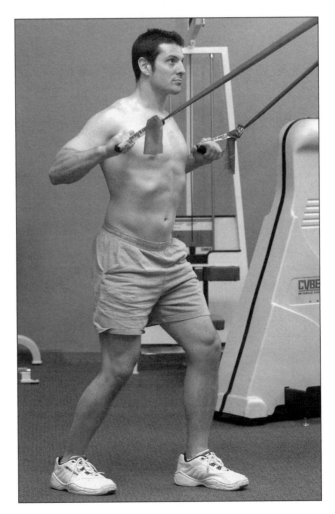

a

Core Emphasis

Sit on exercise ball while performing lat pulldown *(b)*.

Training Tips

Keep back straight and abdominals tight. Keep wrists straight.

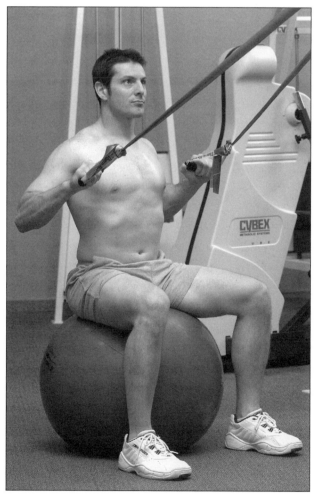

b

SHRUG (Upper Trapezius)

Stand on middle of a long band. Cross bands, and grasp handles at hip level. Shrug shoulders upward *(a)*. Slowly return.

Variation

Upright Row: Begin with elbows straight at hip level, and bend elbows, pulling handles to chest level.

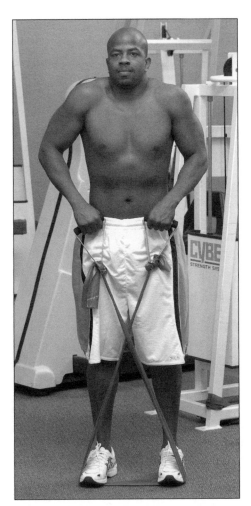

a

Core Emphasis

Stand on one leg while performing upright row exercise. Stand on a foam surface for more challenge *(b)*.

Training Tips

Keep back straight and abdominals tight. Do not arch neck.

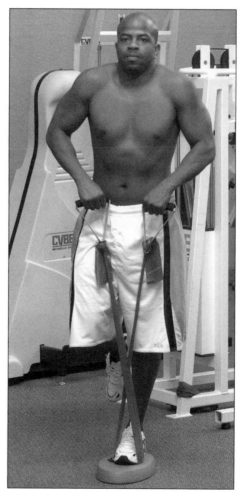

b

BENT-OVER ROW (Rhomboids, Middle Trapezius)

Use staggered step, one leg in front of the other. Stand on middle of band with front foot. Bend forward at hips, keeping back straight. Grasp handles with elbows straight. Pull bands upward by bending elbows, bringing hands to trunk (a). Slowly return.

Variation

Alternate left and right arms while performing bent-over row exercise.

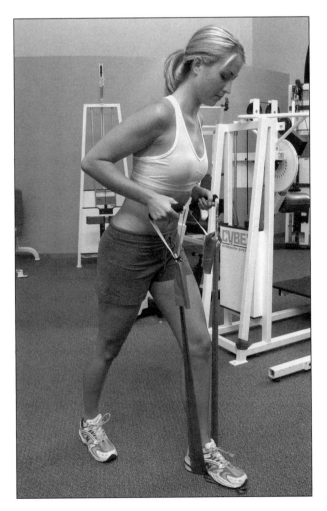

a

Core Emphasis

Stand on front leg while performing bent-over row with right or left arm *(b)*. Stand on a foam surface for more challenge.

Training Tips

Keep back straight. Don't arch neck. Keep wrists straight.

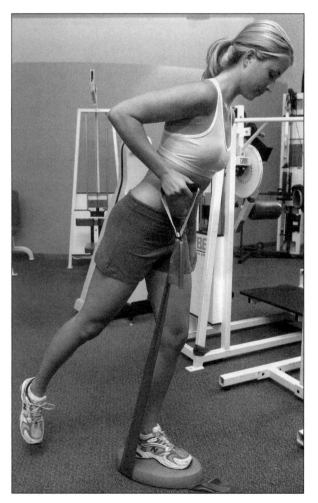

b

CHEST PULLOVER (Pectoralis and Latissimus Dorsi)

Securely attach middle of band to stationary object near floor. Lie on back with knees bent and extend arms overhead. Grasp handles with elbows straight. Keep elbows straight and pull bands down to hips *(a)*. Slowly return.

Variation

Securely attach middle of band to stationary object overhead. While sitting, face away from attachment and extend arms overhead. Grasp handles with elbows straight. Keep elbows straight and pull bands down to hips. Slowly return.

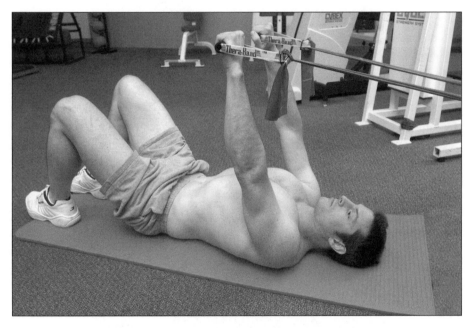

a

Core Emphasis

Lie on exercise ball in a bridge position while performing chest pullover exercise *(b)*.

Training Tips

Keep back straight. Keep elbows and wrists straight.

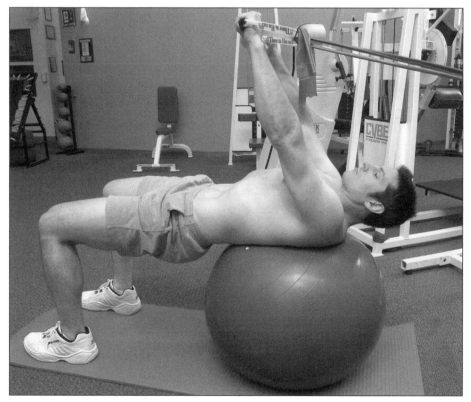

b

PUSH-UP (Pectoralis and Triceps)

Assume push-up position on floor. Stabilize each end of band under a hand, and stretch middle of band across shoulder blades (a). Slowly lower body to floor by bending elbows.

Variation

Perform push-up on toes or knees.

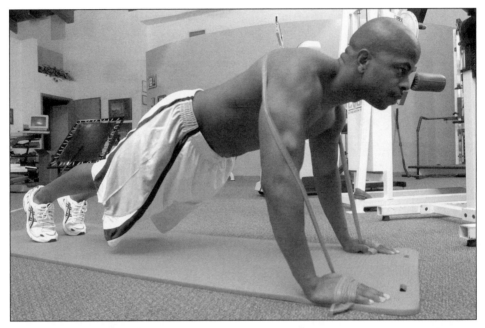

a

Core Emphasis

Place knees or hips on exercise ball while performing push-up *(b)*.

Training Tip

Keep back straight. Don't sag hips.

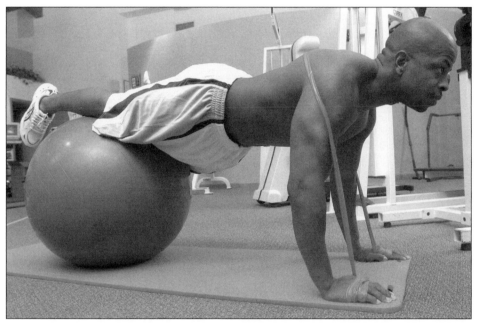

b

DIP (Lower Trapezius and Triceps)

Sit in chair with hands on edge of seat. Secure each end of band under a hand, and stretch middle of band across shoulder blades and behind neck. Keep elbows straight. Scoot forward, lowering hips off chair and keeping feet stationary (a). Press back up against the resistance of band, keeping elbows straight.

Variation

Overhead Dip: Securely attach middle of band to a stationary object overhead. Use a staggered step, one foot slightly in front of other. Grasp the handles with elbows straight, and push downward. Hold. Slowly return.

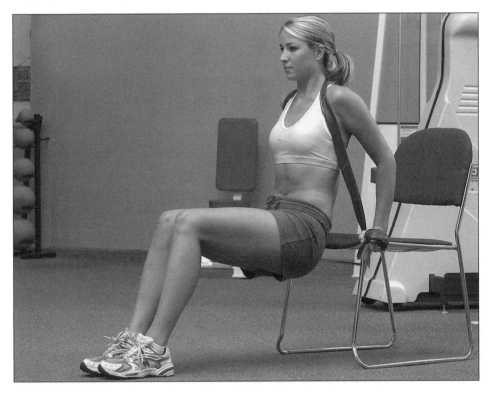

a

Core Emphasis

Perform seated dip with legs and knees extended forward *(b)*.

Training Tip

Keep back straight and abdominals tight.

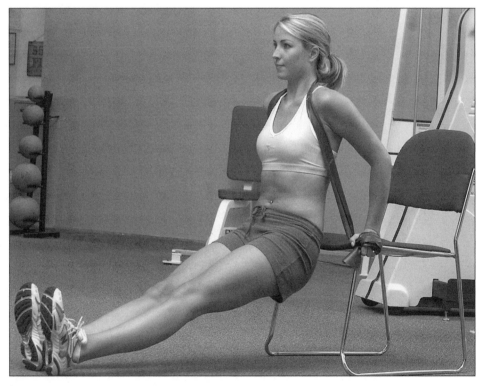

b

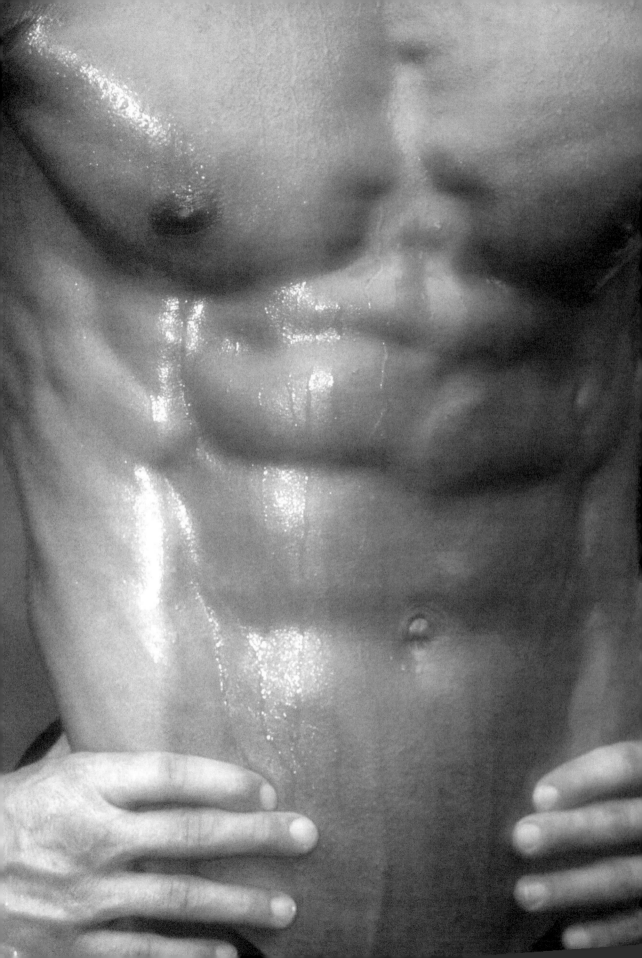

Chapter 4......................

Abdominals and Lower Back

Body-weight resistance is the most common way to strengthen the abdominals and lower-back muscles. Adding external resistance such as an elastic band may increase the training stimulus to these areas, particularly in programs when progress has stalled. The abdominal and core region is a key area for whole-body stabilization and sports performance, most likely because of its ability to generate or transmit forces between the lower extremities and upper extremities. All functional activities of the extremities have some contribution of the core in terms of force production or stabilization. Therefore, core strengthening enhances performance in all sports and functional activities. In addition, strengthening the abdominal and lower-back regions can prevent and improve lower-back pain.

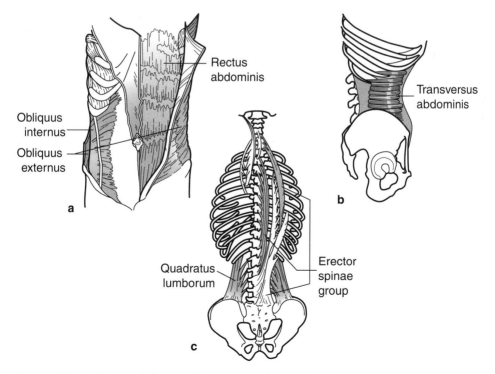

Figure 4.1   *(a)* Rectus abdominis, *(b)* transverse abdominis, *(c)* erector spinae.

CURL-UP (Abdominals)

Securely attach middle of band to stationary object near floor. Lie on back with knees bent, and extend arms in front. Grasp handle with hands close together. Keep elbows straight and curl trunk upward without moving arms. Lift shoulder blades off floor *(a)*. Slowly return.

Variation

Extend arms overhead. Pull arms down toward sides while simultaneously performing curl-up.

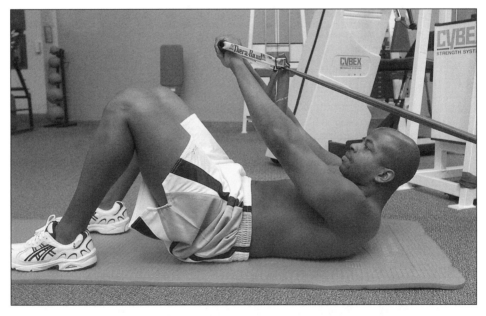

a

Core Emphasis

Lie on an exercise ball in bridge position while performing curl-up exercise *(b)*.

Training Tips

Keep neck straight. Don't protract head. Keep elbows straight.

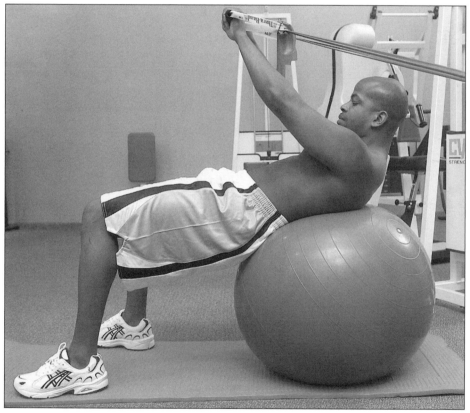

b

LOWER-ABDOMINAL CRUNCH
(Lower Abdominals)

Lie on back with hips and knees flexed. Stretch band over knees and cross underneath. Grasp each end of band on floor at hips, elbows extended by sides. Lift knees upward, lifting hips off floor against resistance of band (a). Slowly return.

Variation

Perform lower-ab crunch with knees straight and legs pointing toward ceiling. Stretch band around feet and push legs upward, lifting hips off floor.

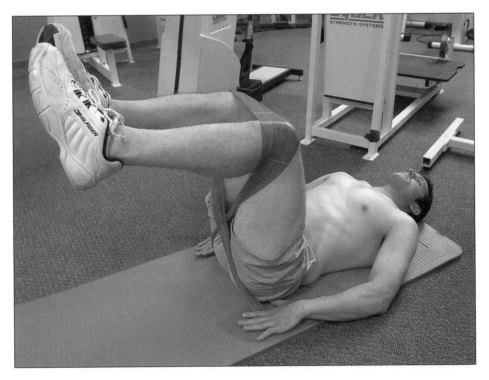

a

Core Emphasis

Lie with knees bent and feet on exercise ball while performing lower-ab crunch exercise *(b)*.

Training Tip

Don't arch the back or flex hips.

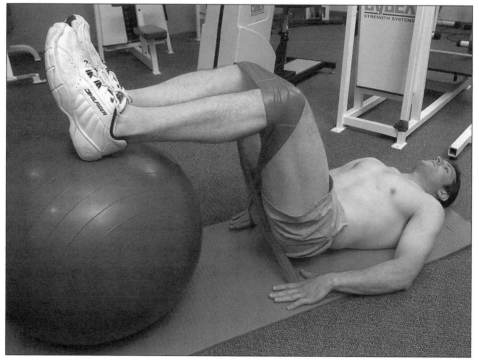

b

TRUNK TWIST (Obliques)

Sit with legs extended at least shoulder-width apart. Stretch middle of band around both feet. Grasp both ends of band with arms extended forward. Rotate trunk to one side *(a)*. Slowly return to other side.

Variation

Securely attach one end of band to stationary object at chest level. Stand in athletic stance with knees and hips slightly bent and back straight. Grasp other end of band with arms extended forward. Rotate trunk to one side *(b)*. Slowly return.

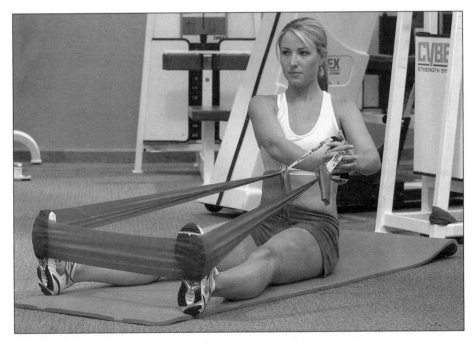

a

Core Emphasis

Stand on one leg while performing oblique twist exercise variation. Stand on a foam surface for more challenge *(b)*.

Training Tip

Keep back straight. Don't lean to one side.

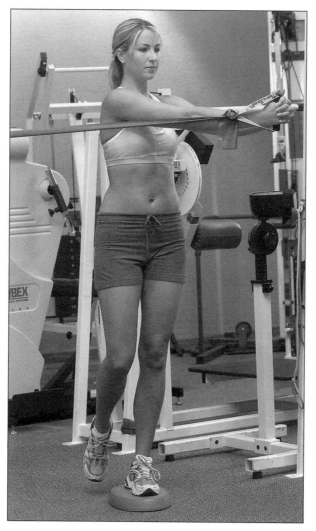

b

BACK EXTENSION (Multifidus)

Sit with legs extended. Stretch middle of band around both feet. Grasp both ends of band with hands at chest. Lean back, stretching the band (a). Keep lumbar spine (lower back) straight. Slowly return.

Variation

Perform sitting back extension with elbows straight.

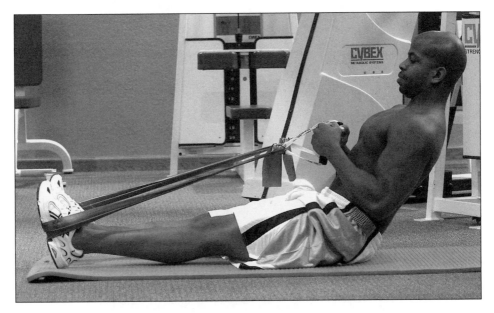

a

Core Emphasis

Stand in a lunge position with middle of band under front foot. Grasp ends of band, and keep elbows bent *(b)*. Extend back and hips against band. Keep spine straight. Stand on foam surface for more challenge.

Training Tip

Keep lumbar spine in "neutral" position; not too rounded or hyperextended.

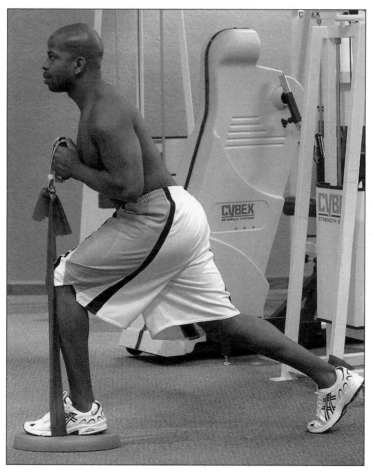

b

SIDE BEND (Quadratus Lumborum)

Stand with feet shoulder-width apart, knees and hips slightly bent, and back straight. Grasp one end of band and extend arm overhead. Lean trunk away from band, stretching band. Slowly return.

Variation

Stand on the middle of band and grasp one end by your side. Keeping elbow straight, grasp other end of band. Lean trunk away from band, stretching band (a).

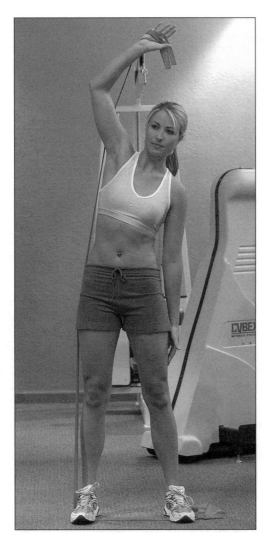

a

Core Emphasis

Stand on one leg while performing overhead side-bend exercise. Stand on a foam surface for more challenge *(b)*.

Training Tip

Keep trunk aligned. Don't rotate trunk or shift hips.

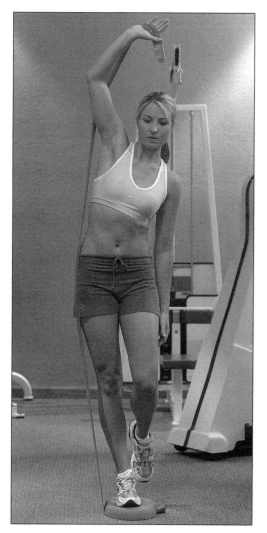

b

SIDE BRIDGE (Quadratus Lumborum)

Lie on side with band wrapped around knees. Bend elbow and place under shoulder closest to the floor. Keep knees bent, and lift hips off floor with back straight *(a)*. Hold this position and separate knees, stretching band. Slowly return.

Variation

Perform side bridge exercise with knees straight, bridging from feet.

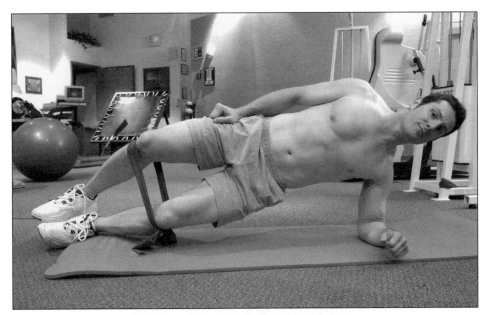

a

Core Emphasis

Grasp one end of band in stabilizing hand on floor, and other end in other hand. Perform exercise with knees straight. Keep elbow straight while stretching band toward ceiling *(b)*. Slowly return.

Training Tip

Keep hips and spine aligned. Don't drop hips or rotate trunk.

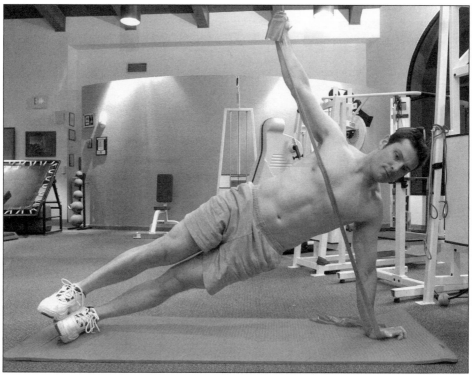

b

BRIDGE (Gluteus Maximus)

Lie on back with middle of band stretched around waist and crossed behind, underneath buttocks. Grasp each end of band with hands placed under shoulders. Lift buttocks off floor with knees bent and elbows extended, stretching band (a). Slowly return.

Variation

While in the bridge position with band stretched, march knees by alternately lifting them up and down.

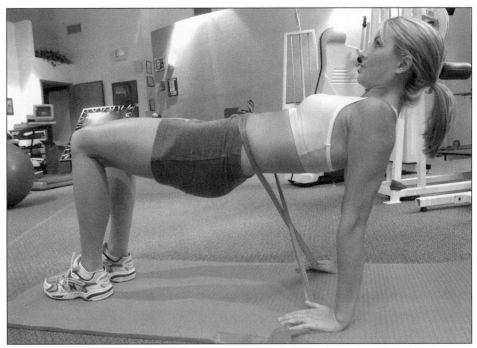

a

Core Emphasis

Place feet across exercise ball while performing bridging exercise. Stabilize ends of band with hands by hips *(b)*.

Training Tip

Keep hips level at top of bridge. Don't let hips or back sag.

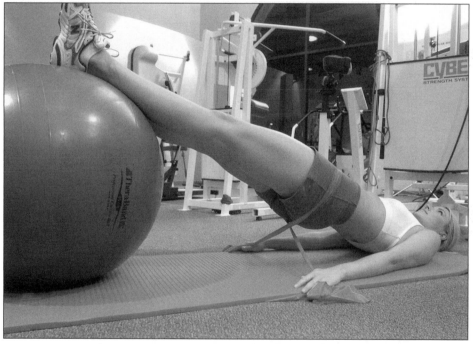

b

LIFT (Posterior Trunk and Shoulder)

Securely attach one end of band to stationary object near floor. Begin in an athletic stance, hips and knees slightly bent. Stand to side of attachment. Grasp handle with both hands, and slightly rotate trunk toward band. Lift band over opposite shoulder with both hands, turning trunk away from attachment (a). Slowly return.

Variation

Add more rotation, side bending, or flexion of trunk to lifting movement.

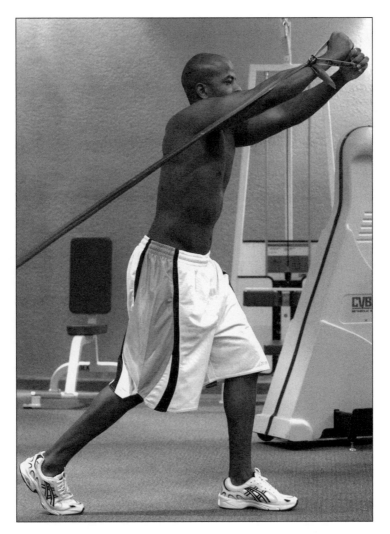

a

Core Emphasis

Stand on one leg while performing the lifting exercise. Stand on a foam surface for more challenge *(b)*.

Training Tip

Keep back in neutral position at top of movement. Don't arch the back.

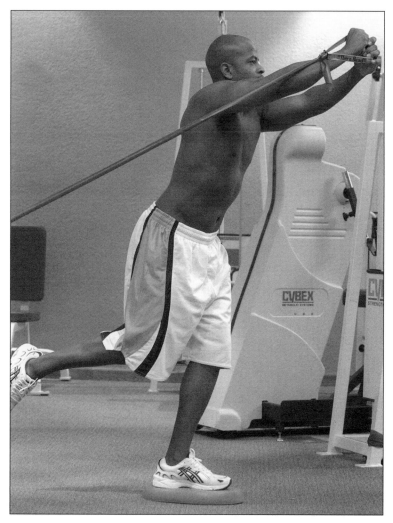

b

CHOP (Anterior Trunk and Shoulder)

Securely attach one end of band to stationary object overhead. Begin in an athletic stance, hips and knees slightly bent. Grasp handle with both hands over shoulder closest to attachment, with trunk slightly rotated toward band. Pull band down to opposite hip with both hands, turning trunk away from attachment (a). Slowly return.

Variation

Add more rotation, side bending, or flexion of trunk to chopping movement.

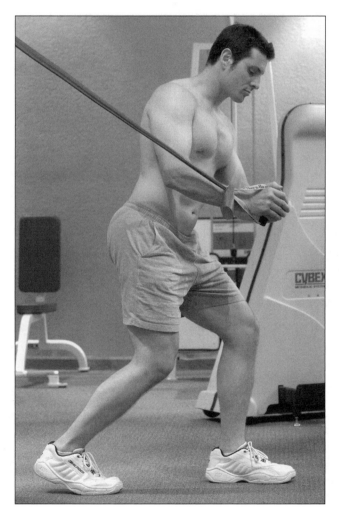

a

Core Emphasis

Stand on one leg while performing chopping exercise. Stand on a foam surface for more challenge *(b)*.

Training Tip

Keep back in neutral position at top of movement. Don't round back.

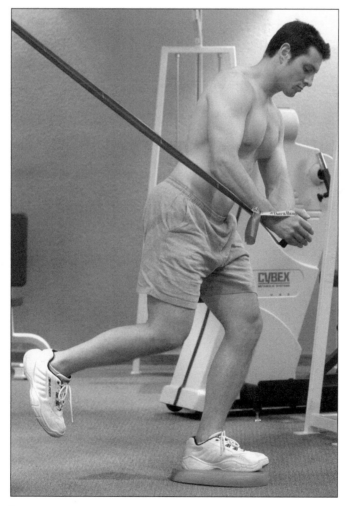

b

QUADRUPED STABILIZATION (Lumbar Stabilizers)

Assume a quadruped position, on hands and knees. Wrap middle of band around sole of one foot, and stabilize ends of band in both hands. Keeping back and neck straight, extend leg backward against band until parallel to floor (a). Slowly return.

Variation

Perform hip extension against band simultaneously with one-arm flexion.

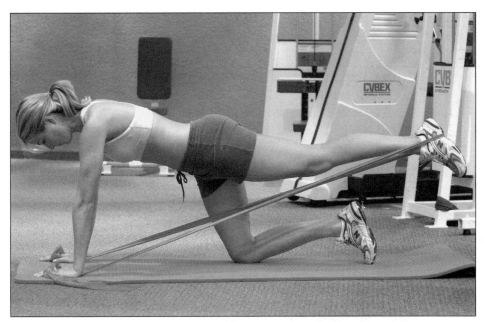

a

Core Emphasis

Grasp one end of band in stabilizing hand on floor, and other end in other hand. Perform exercise with knees straight. Keep elbow straight while stretching band toward ceiling *(b)*. Slowly return.

Training Tip

Keep hips and spine aligned. Don't drop hips or rotate trunk.

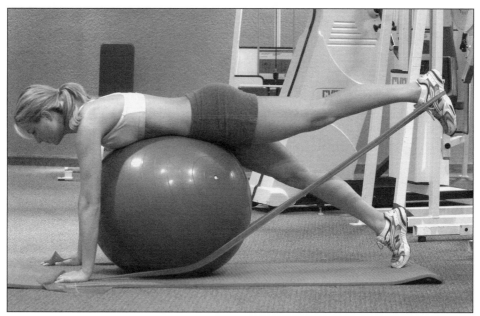

b

SUPINE STABILIZATION (Lumbar Stabilizers)

Lie on back with one leg straight and the other flexed. Wrap middle of band around sole of foot of straight leg, and grasp other ends of band, elbows extended upward *(a)*. Alternate flexing arms with elbows straight. Keep back straight. Slowly return.

Variation

Perform hip flexion and extension (knee straight) against band simultaneously with one-arm flexion.

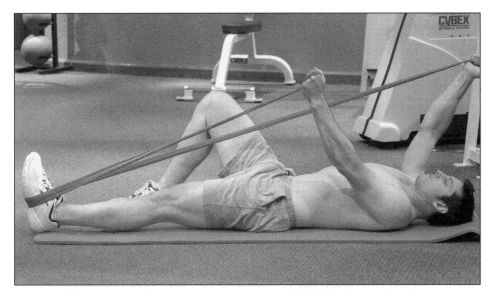

a

Core Emphasis

Stand while performing alternating hip extension and arm flexion. Stand on a foam surface for more challenge *(b)*.

Training Tip

Keep back and neck straight in neutral position. Don't arch the back.

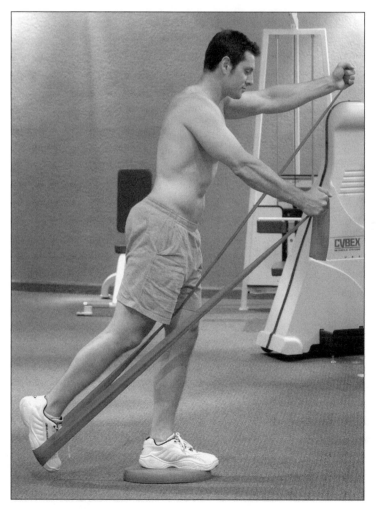

b

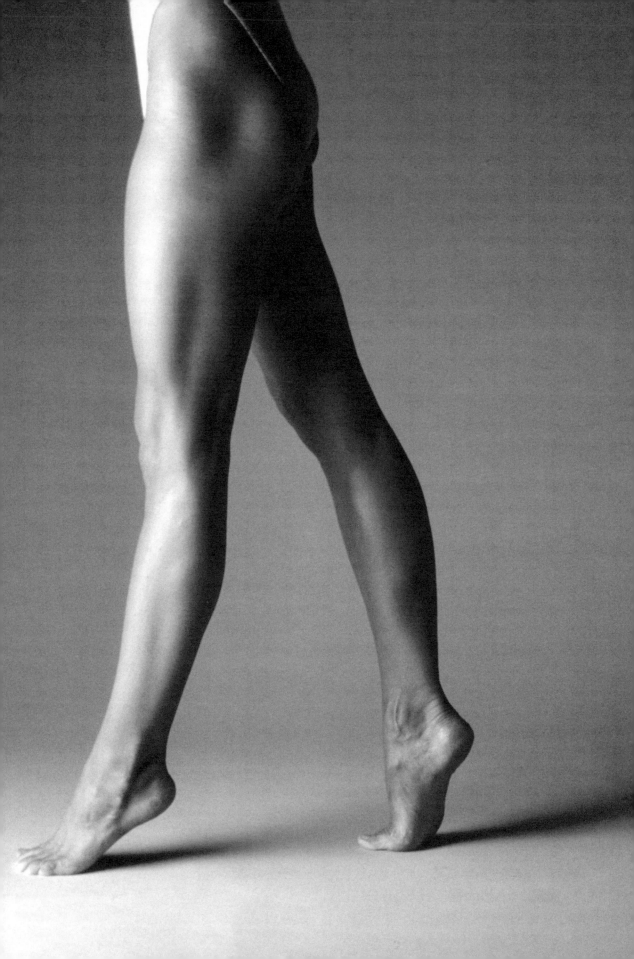

Chapter 5..............................
Hips and Thighs

One of the most important areas of the body to strengthen is the hip and thigh region. As the main link between the lower extremities and the trunk, the hips serve as a stable base for the "core" (the abdominals and lower-back region). The hips perform the main role in locomotion, moving our centers of gravity in walking and running. The gluteal muscles (gluteus maximus and medius) are also important pelvic stabilizers. Therefore, the hips and the core are linked in a kinetic chain to transmit and produce force throughout the body. Strong hip muscles are vital to daily activities, particularly during walking or running. In fact, weakness of the gluteal muscles has been linked to chronic back pain and even repetitive ankle sprains. Another role of the hip and thigh musculature is to "decelerate," or slow down motion, or to change direction of motion. This specialized muscle activity (which often goes untrained) may be a cause of repetitive hip flexor, groin, and hamstring strains in athletes. Finally, an imbalance of strength and flexibility between the quadriceps and hamstrings muscles has been linked to knee pain and injury. It's important to remember that the core emphasis exercises should be performed with slightly less resistance than the basic exercises.

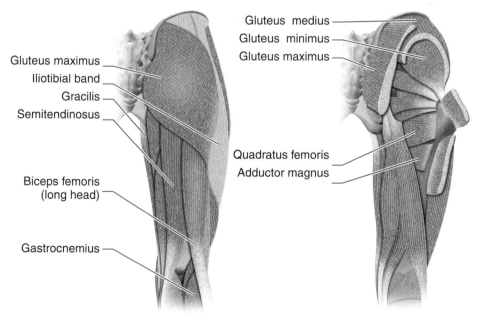

Figure 5.1 Hip and thigh muscles.

HIP FLEXION (Iliopsoas)

Sit on exercise ball or chair. Secure both ends of band under one foot. Loop middle of band around thigh of other leg *(a)*. Lift hip. Slowly return.

Variation

Secure both ends of band to stationary object near floor. Loop middle of band around ankle. Face away from attachment, and kick leg forward, keeping knee straight.

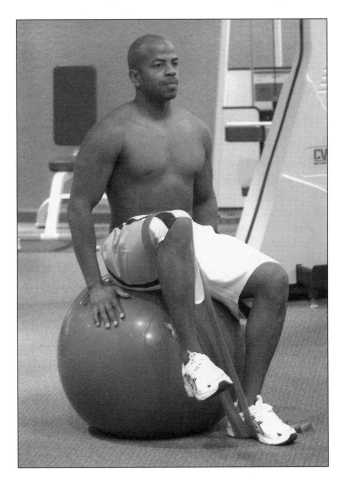

a

Core Emphasis

Stand with both ends of band under one foot. Loop middle of band around lower thigh of opposite leg. While balancing on leg securing the band, lift opposite knee upward to hip level, stretching band *(b)*. Slowly return. Stand on a foam surface for more challenge.

Training Tips

Keep back straight. Keep abdominals tight.

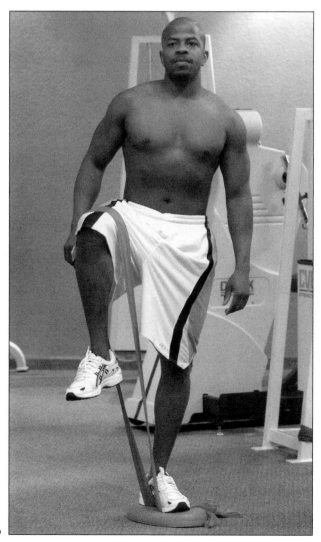

b

HIP EXTENSION (Gluteus Maximus)

Assume a quadruped position, on hands and knees. Rest on elbows, keeping back straight. Secure both ends of band under forearms, and loop middle of band around one foot. Keep knee bent and extend hip upward against band (a). Slowly return.

Variation

Secure both ends of band to stationary object near floor. Loop middle of band around ankle. Face attachment. Kick leg backward, keeping knee straight.

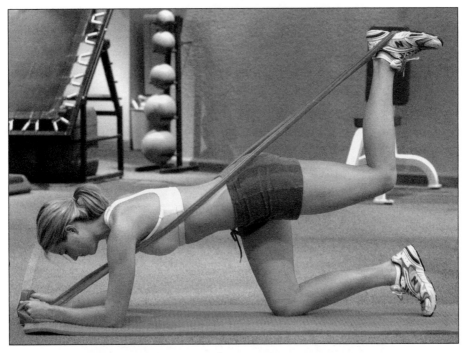

a

Core Emphasis

Loop middle of band around knee, and secure both ends of band to stationary object. Face attachment. Kick leg backward, keeping knee bent *(b)*. Stand on a foam surface for more challenge.

Training Tips

Keep back straight. Keep abdominals tight.

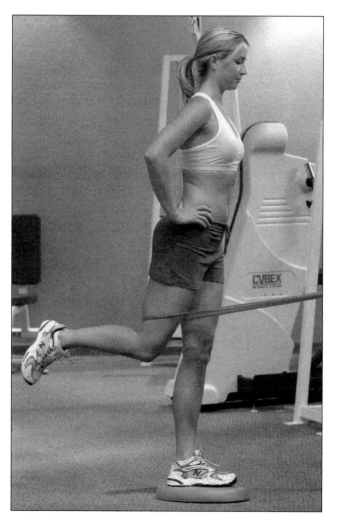

b

HIP ABDUCTION (Gluteus Medius)

Sit with legs extended and band looped around both ankles. Lean back onto elbows in a reclining position (a). Keeping one leg stationary, push the other leg outward, keeping knee straight. Slowly return.

Variation

Secure both ends of band to stationary object near the floor. With side you are exercising farthest from the attachment, loop middle of band around ankle of one leg. With that leg, kick outward, keeping knee straight.

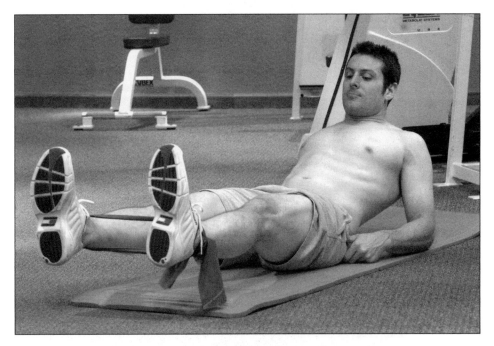

a

Core Emphasis

Stand on middle of band. Grasp both ends at hip level. Stand on one leg, and kick other leg outward *(b)*. Keep knees straight. Slowly return. Stand on a foam surface for more challenge.

Training Tips

Keep back straight. Don't shift hips. Keep abdominals tight.

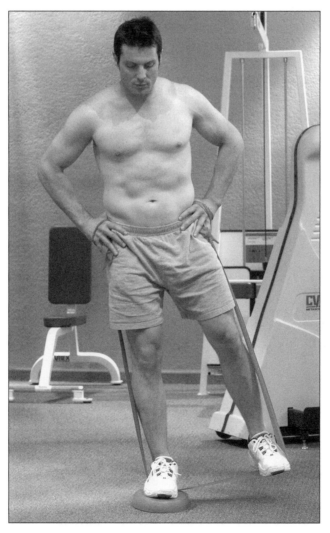

b

HIP INTERNAL AND EXTERNAL ROTATION
(Hip Rotators)

Secure both ends of band to stationary object near floor. Loop middle of band around ankle. In a half-kneeling position (one knee up), rotate lower leg away from attachment, stretching band. Slowly return. For external rotation, exercising leg should be closest to attachment *(a)*. For internal rotation, exercising leg should be farthest from the attachment *(b)*.

Variation

Sit in chair to perform hip internal or external rotation. Secure both ends of band to stationary object. Loop middle of band around ankle and rotate lower leg, stretching band.

Core Emphasis

Wrap middle of band around hips. Grasp each end of band. Stand on leg to be exercised and extend arm on opposite side forward, stretching

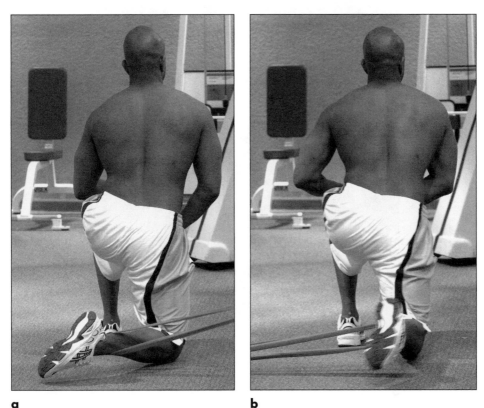

a   **b**

band. Keep other hand at waist *(c)*. Twist hip of stance leg, pushing hip of opposite leg backward into band. Slowly return. Stand on a foam surface for more challenge.

Training Tips

Keep back straight. Don't bend hip.

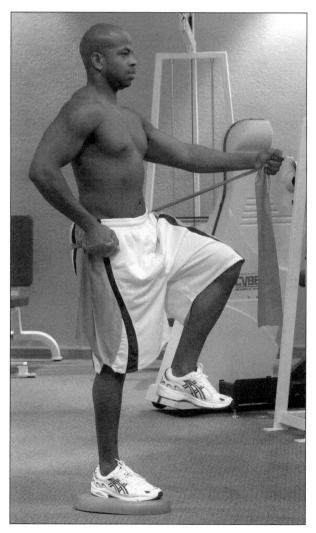

c

KNEE EXTENSION (Quadriceps)

Secure both ends of band to stationary object about knee level. Wrap middle of band around ankle. Lie on stomach with head next to attachment. Bend knee of exercising leg *(a)*. Extend knee, stretching band, until it reaches floor. Slowly return.

Variation

Sit in chair to perform knee extension. Secure both ends of band to stationary object. Face away from attachment. Wrap middle of band around ankle. Extend knee. Slowly return.

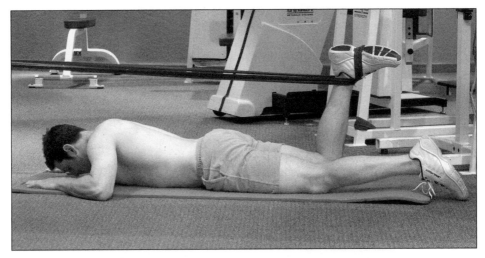

a

Core Emphasis

Stand with both ends of band under one foot. Wrap middle of band around ankle of opposite leg. Stand on leg securing band. Lift opposite knee upward to hip level, stretching band, then extend knee forward *(b)*. Slowly return. Stand on a foam surface for more challenge.

Training Tip

Keep back straight and abdominals tight.

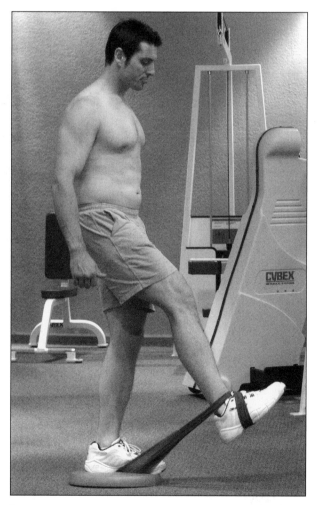

b

KNEE FLEXION (Hamstrings)

Secure both ends of band to stationary object about knee height. Wrap middle of band around ankle. Lie on stomach with head away from attachment. Bend knee of exercising leg *(a)*, stretching band and pulling it toward buttocks. Slowly return.

Variation

Sit in chair to perform knee flexion. Secure both ends of band to stationary object. Face attachment. Wrap middle of band around ankle. Flex knee. Slowly return.

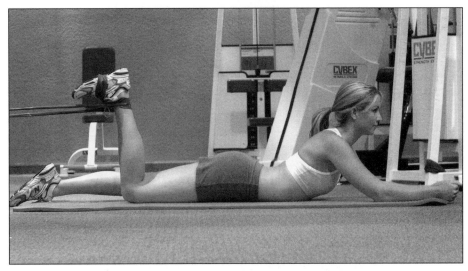

a

Core Emphasis

Stand with both ends of band under one foot. Wrap middle of band around ankle. Stand on the exercising leg. Slightly extend hip, stretching band, then flex knee, lifting band upward *(b)*. Slowly return. Stand on a foam surface for more challenge.

Training Tip

Keep back straight and abdominals tight.

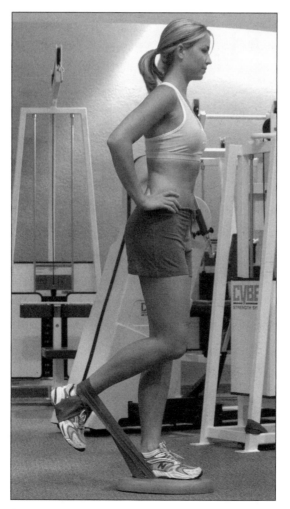

b

LEG PRESS (Gluteus Maximus and Quadriceps)

Lie with knees bent and middle of band looped around sole of one foot. Grasp ends of band *(a)*. Extend hip and knee against band until straight. Slowly return.

Variation

Loop middle of band around one foot. Assume a quadruped position, on hands and knees, keeping back straight. Grasp each end of band. Extend hip and knee of exercising leg against band until leg is even with trunk. Slowly return.

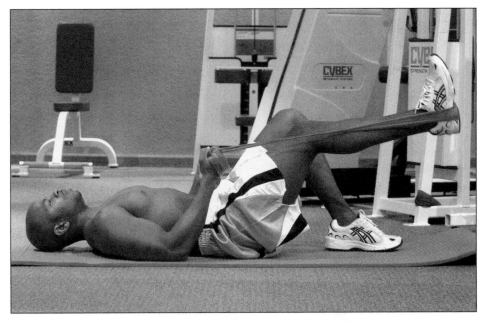

a

Core Emphasis

Recline on exercise ball. Place one leg on floor for stability. Loop middle of band around foot. Grasp ends. Extend hip and knee until straight *(b)*. Slowly return.

Training Tip
Keep back straight and abdominals tight.

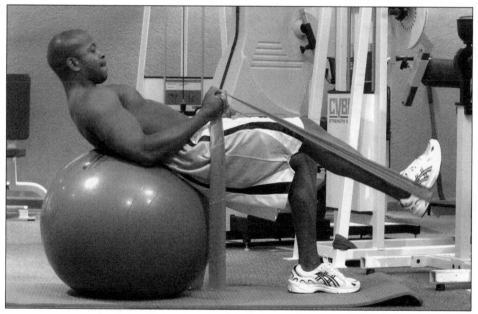

b

SQUAT (Gluteus Maximus and Quadriceps)

Stand on middle of long band. Bring band around outside of feet. Cross band behind knees and bring both ends around to front. Grasp ends, keeping hands at hip level *(a)*. Perform squat, keeping back straight. Slowly return.

Variation

Stand on middle of long band. Bring band around outside of feet. Grasp ends, keeping hands at hip or shoulder level. Perform squat, keeping back straight.

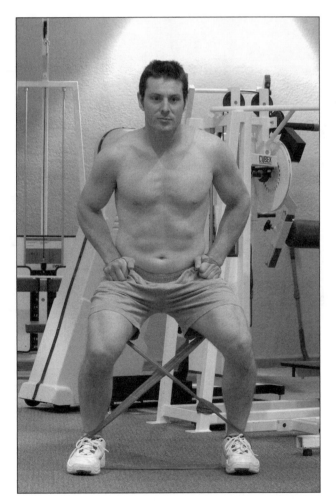

a

Core Emphasis

Perform squat exercise with bands crossed while simultaneously performing diagonal flexion exercise with both shoulders *(b)*. Stand on a foam surface for more challenge.

Training Tip

Keep back straight and abdominals tight.

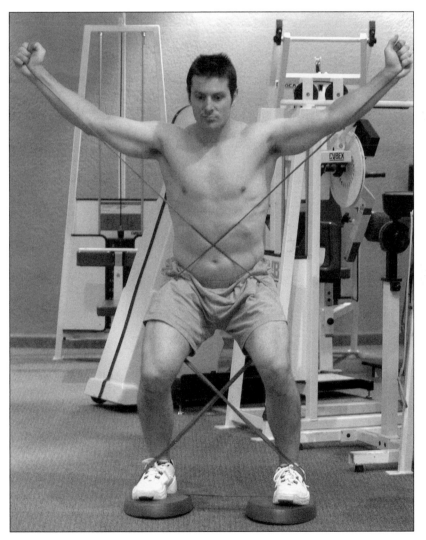

b

LUNGE (Gluteus Maximus and Quadriceps)

Stand with one foot on middle of band. Grasp ends, keeping hands at hip level with elbows bent. Place other leg behind with knee bent (a). Keeping trunk upright, bend front knee, lowering the body. Slowly return.

Variation

Perform lunge exercise with band held at shoulder level.

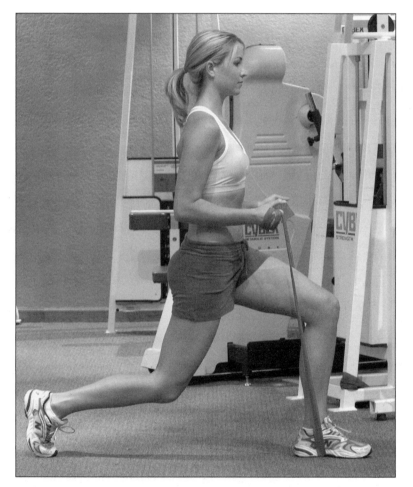

a

Core Emphasis

Perform lunge exercise with band while simultaneously performing diagonal flexion exercise with both shoulders *(b)*. Stand on a foam surface for more challenge.

Training Tips

Keep back straight and abdominals tight. Keep trunk upright at all times.

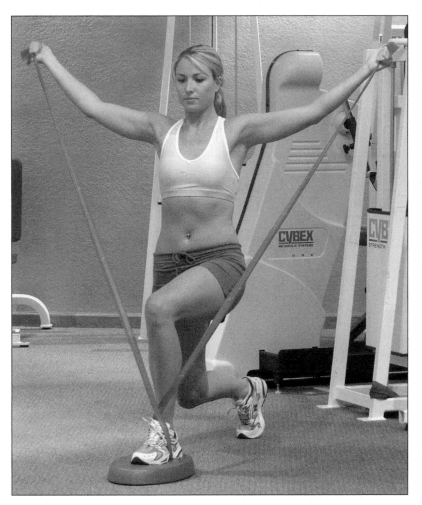

b

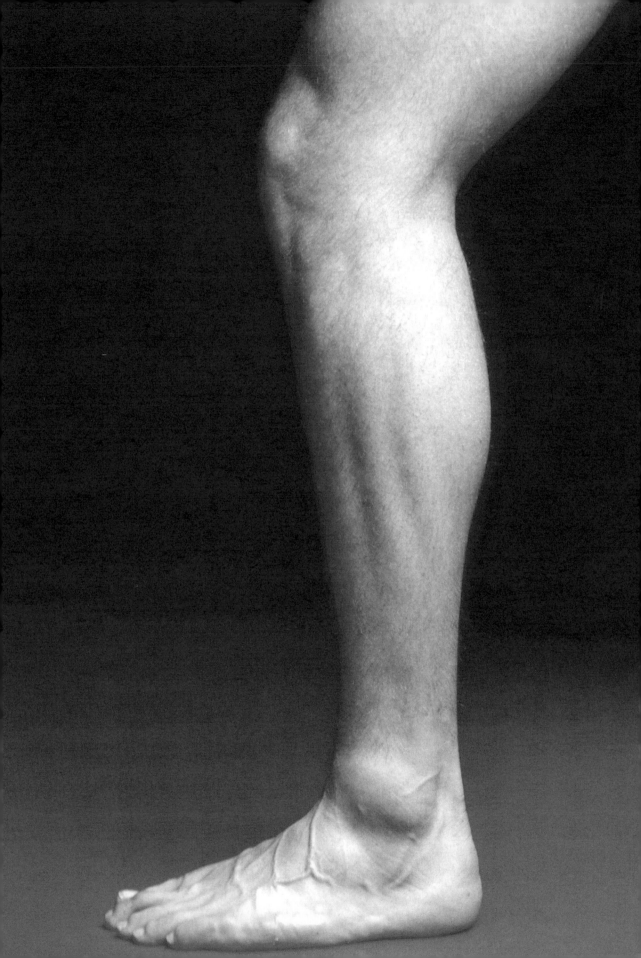

Chapter 6..........................
Lower Legs and Ankles

The lower leg and ankle musculature is difficult to exercise with traditional weight-training equipment. Because of the smaller ranges of motion used with ankle exercise, elastic resistance is ideal for strengthening the lower leg. The anterior and posterior muscles (tibialis anterior, and gastrocnemius and soleus muscles, respectively) have important roles in gait and locomotion, whereas the medial (tibialis posterior) and lateral (peroneus longus) muscles perform important stabilizing roles. ERT of the ankle is often used to rehabilitate or prevent ankle sprains. Ankle sprains are more common in football, soccer, basketball, and tennis players, because of quick changes in direction. The core emphasis exercises should be performed with slightly less resistance than in the basic exercises.

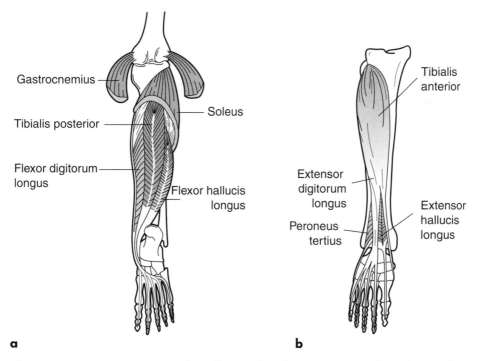

Figure 6.1 *(a)* Extrinsic posterior lower leg muscles, *(b)* extrinsic anterior lower leg muscles.

DORSIFLEXION (Tibialis Anterior)

Sit on floor with both knees extended. Loop middle of band around one foot. Grasp ends of band in opposite hand and push down on band with other foot. Lift foot of ankle being exercised against resistance of band *(a)*. Slowly return.

Variation

Perform exercise while sitting with knees bent. Loop middle of band around one foot and stabilize band under other foot *(b)*. Lift foot of ankle being exercised upward. Slowly return.

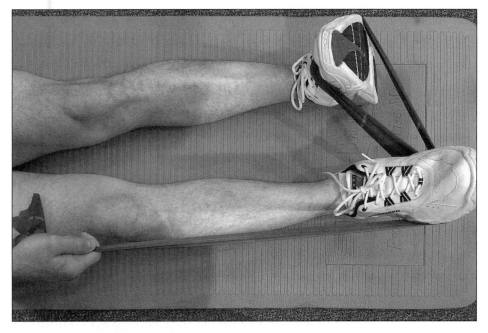

a

Core Emphasis

Sit on exercise ball while performing dorsiflexion *(b)*.

Training Tip

Keep knee from moving excessively to complete exercise.

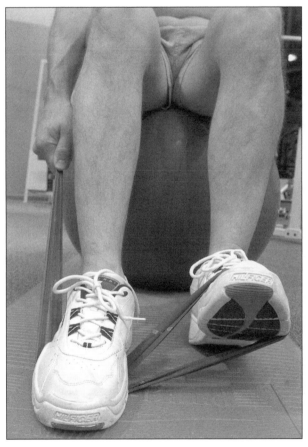

b

PLANTAR FLEXION (Gastrocnemius and Soleus)

Sit on floor with both knees extended. Loop middle of band around one foot. Grasp ends of band. Push foot down against resistance of band (a). Slowly return.

Variation

Perform exercise while sitting with knees bent (to isolate soleus muscle). Loop middle of band under foot placed on floor. Stabilize ends of band across knee. Push foot down into floor, lifting heel against resistance of band (b). Slowly return.

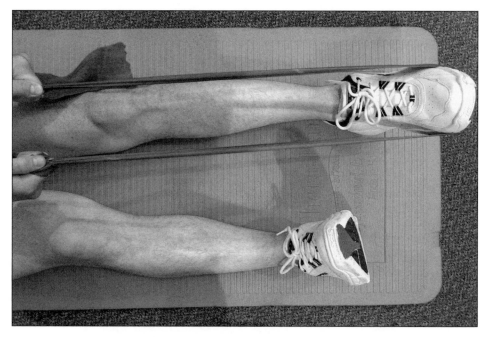

a

Core Emphasis

Sit on exercise ball with knees bent (to isolate soleus muscle).

Training Tip

Keep knee from moving excessively to complete exercise.

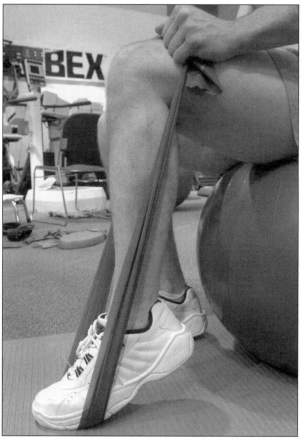

b

INVERSION (Tibialis Posterior)

Sit on floor with opposite knee on top of leg to be exercised. Loop middle of band around foot to be exercised. Wrap bands around opposite foot and grasp ends of band. Turn foot inward against resistance of the band *(a)*. Slowly return.

Variation

Sit with foot being exercised across opposite knee. Loop middle of band around foot, and secure ends of band under opposite foot *(b)*. Lift foot being exercised. Slowly return.

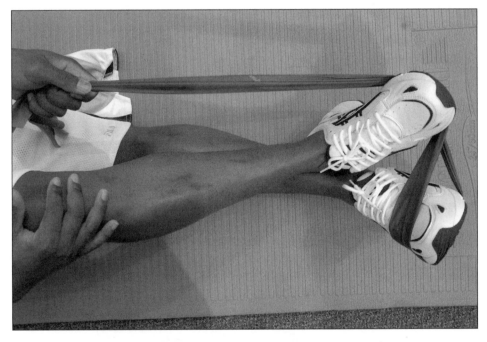

a

Core Emphasis

Sit on exercise ball while performing the sitting variation exercise *(b)*.

Training Tip

Keep knee and hip stable. Don't rotate leg to complete exercise.

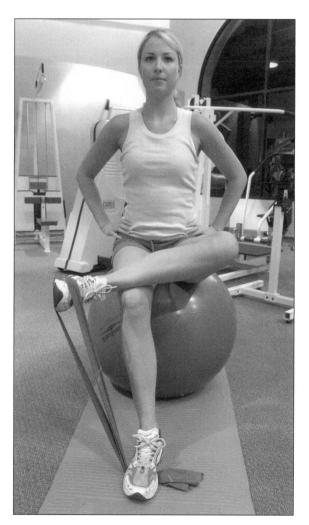

b

EVERSION (Peroneus longus)

Sit on floor with both knees extended. Loop middle of band around one foot, and wrap ends over opposite foot. Grasp ends of band in opposite hand *(a)*. Turn foot outward, away from band. Slowly return.

Variation

Sit with knees bent and middle of band looped around foot being exercised. Secure ends of band under opposite foot. Turn foot outward, away from band *(b)*. Slowly return.

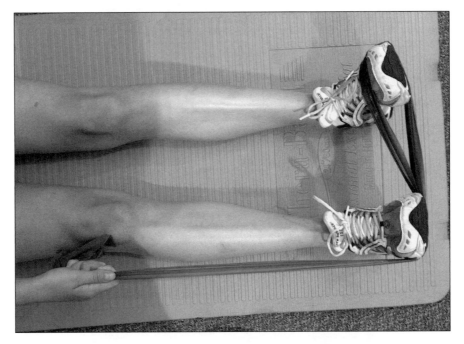

a

Core Emphasis

Sit on exercise ball while performing the sitting variation exercise.

Training Tip

Keep knee and hip stable. Don't rotate leg to complete exercise.

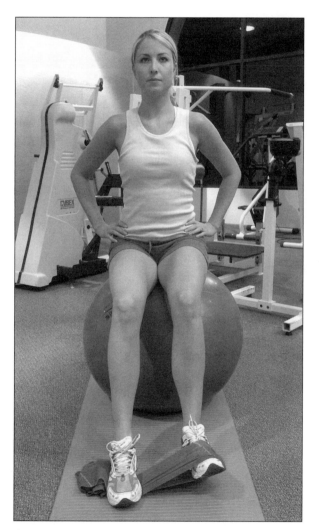

b

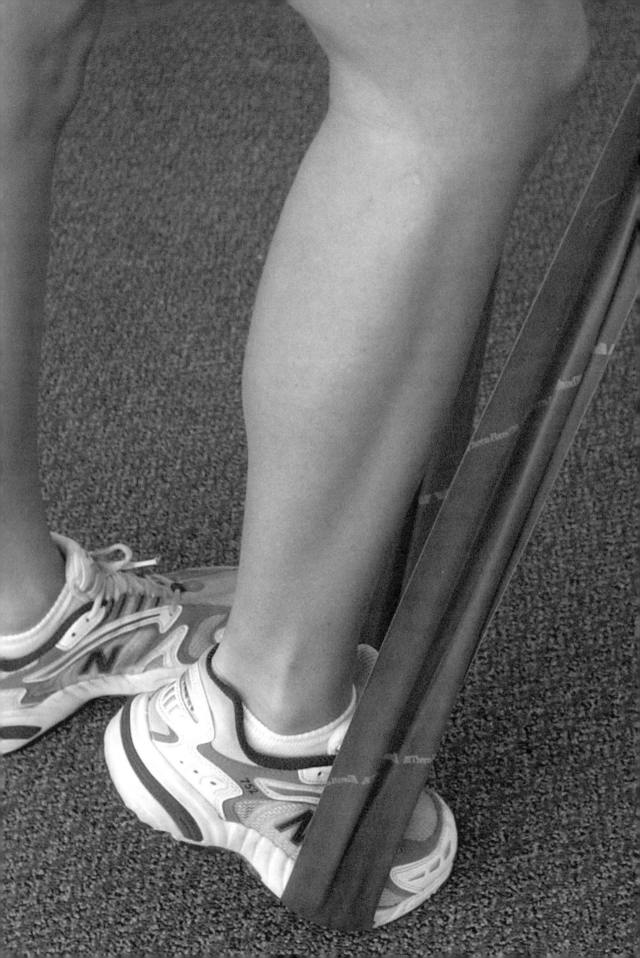

Chapter 7...........................

Combination and Circuit Training

Elastic resistance is quickly becoming one of the most popular forms of fitness resistance training. While therapists have used elastic resistance training predominantly for rehabilitation, fitness and sports trainers are finding elastic resistance to be a valuable tool to complement traditional strength-training routines. Incorporating elastic resistance training into traditional weight-training routines helps prevent "staleness" of the routine, and also allows for additional exercises that may not be possible with isotonic resistance. In addition, elastic resistance can "isolate" certain muscles (such as the rotator cuff) with a resistance lower than that possible on multijoint machines. Further, elastic resistance enables the easy replication of sport-specific movements (see chapter 10).

The versatility of elastic bands and tubing means they can be used not only for muscle strengthening, but also in combination with other exercise modes, including aerobic, circuit, and aquatic programs. Partnering programs with elastic resistance expands group-strengthening routines as well. Elastic resistance exercise offers more program options that may appeal to a larger number of participants, and its many options may be used to develop "niche" programs targeted to specific populations, such as those suffering osteoarthritis, or in fall-prevention for older adults.

Combination Training

Elastic resistance is an excellent choice to combine with traditional isotonic exercises to add variety to a resistance training program. In chapter 8, we describe how elastic resistance can be combined directly with isotonic resistance for power training; however, specific elastic resistance exercises can be combined within isotonic exercise routines to provide a well-rounded strengthening program. A single piece of band or tubing can provide a variety of exercises that may target a muscle or muscle group slightly differently than resistance machines do. For example, performing a bench press with a barbell is much different from performing the same movement against elastic resistance in a standing position, which is not possible with free weights. In addition, more core strength and stabilization is needed to perform a bench press while standing compared with the traditional bench press, so this increases the efficiency of the exercise. Elastic resistance also allows individuals to strengthen areas difficult to train with machines, such as the rotator cuff and small muscles of the ankle.

Some examples of combination training are as follows:

- Alternate barbell bench press with elastic band bench press (page 36)
- Alternate dumbell lateral raises with elastic band PNF diagonals (pages 22-23)
- Alternate knee extension machine with elastic band standing knee extension kicks (page 91)
- Alternate abdominal curl ups with elastic band lower ab crunches (page 60)

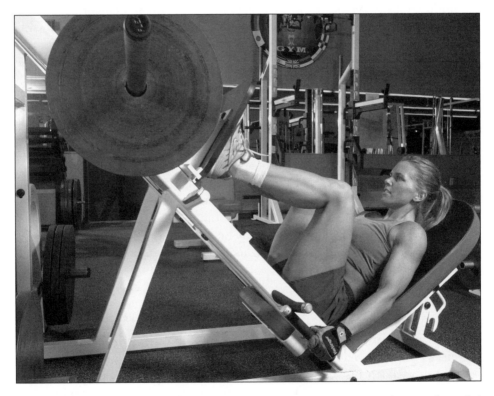

Combining traditional strength training with elastic resistance training provides a well-rounded strengthening program.

Circuit Training

Circuit training is a popular conditioning program that incorporates different "stations" of exercise that are done for a specific length of time. Participants move from station to station, completing each station exercise once or more during the course of the program. This method is quite effective in small group programs, efficiently exercising several people with a limited number of strength-training devices. Well-designed circuit training also facilitates training reciprocal muscle groups, improving muscle balance. By combining traditional isotonic exercises with elastic resistance exercises, exercise professionals can create well-rounded circuit training routines for strength. Elastic bands and tubing can easily be attached to heavy stationary isotonic machines and can quickly and easily be used in the circuit (see figure 7.1). For example, an upper-body strengthening circuit may include:

Station 1: bench-press machine

Station 2: seated-row machine

Station 3: rotator cuff (internal and external) exercise using tubing

Station 4: overhead-press machine

Station 5: lat-pulldown machine

Station 6: PNF diagonals using tubing

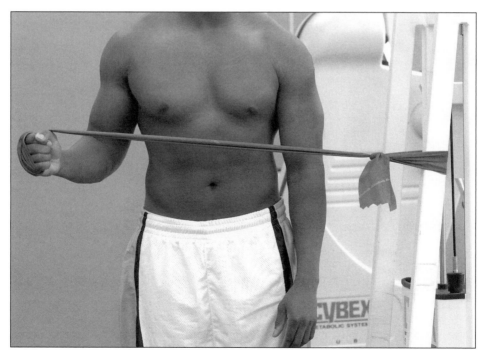

Figure 7.1   Strengthening the rotator cuff using an elastic band by attaching it to a machine.

This circuit is effective for six people to perform exercises on machines and with elastic tubing. For example, each person would have a specific length of time (30 to 60 seconds) to perform a prescribed number of repetitions (10 to 20), and then move to the next station. This rotation would occur two more times, to complete three sets of each exercise.

Group Training

While traditionally used for individualized training, elastic resistance is also popular in larger-group exercise programs. This trend grew out of the need to expand exercise program options in fitness facilities, as well as a need to incorporate strengthening exercises with traditional aerobic conditioning programs. As the population became busier and time to exercise became less, the fitness profession developed new programs to combine strength and cardiovascular workouts to save people time and to use that time more efficiently. Recent research has shown that combining elastic resistance strengthening with traditional aerobic routines improves cardiovascular conditioning more than cardio training alone.

Elastic bands and tubing for group fitness programs is often provided in fixed lengths with handles attached (see figure 7.2). Because they are inexpensive, easy to store, and portable, these elastic devices are ideal for group programs. Incorporating elastic resistance training into traditional programs such as step

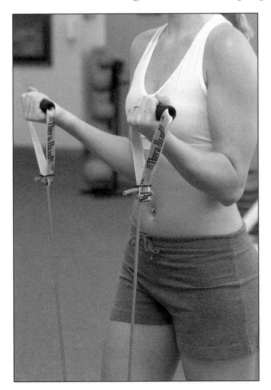

Figure 7.2 Example of using tubing in a fitness program.

aerobics is very easy. Any of the exercises shown in chapters 2 through 6 can be used in a group program set to music. Figure 7.3a-b demonstrates examples of incorporating elastic tubing with step aerobics.

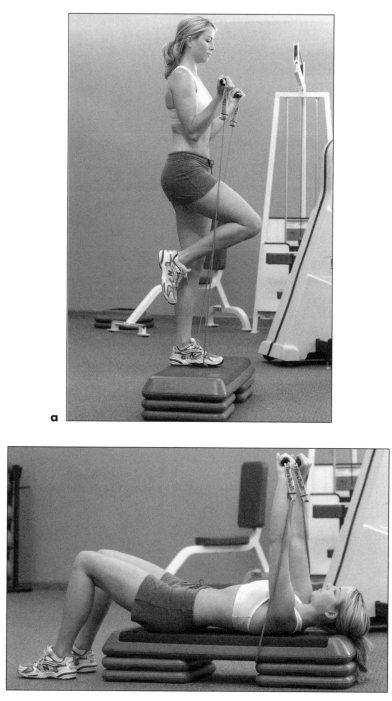

Figure 7.3   *(a)* Using the tube in the step up, *(b)* and with the bench press on a fitness step.

Some common elastic resistance exercises commonly used in group training are as follows:

- Elbow curls (page 26)
- Lateral raises (page 14) and front raises (page 16)
- Overhead press (page 18)

"Toning" classes set to music, which focus on group strengthening routines rather than cardiovascular programs, are also becoming popular. One advantage of elastic resistance strengthening programs in groups is that one band or tubing length can be used for a variety of exercises without the need for various machines or lots of space. Simple changes in resistance level are possible by shortening or lengthening the elastic band or tubing, eliminating the need for a set of dumbbell weights. Finally, there may be less danger of damaging the floor or of injury if dumbbells are not part of the routines.

Partner Training

Using elastic resistance with a partner can expand training options for individuals or groups. By using a partner to hold one end of the band, there's no need to attach it to a stationary object, which is ideal during group training. Both individuals may resist each other's simultaneous movements as well, making a very efficient workout (see figure 7.4a-b). Exercising against a partner requires more balance, coordination, and core strength. In addition, working together builds camaraderie and cooperation. Finally, less equipment is needed since one piece of elastic resistance is used by two people, making it a great "two for one workout." Remember to pair partners of similar strength and ability.

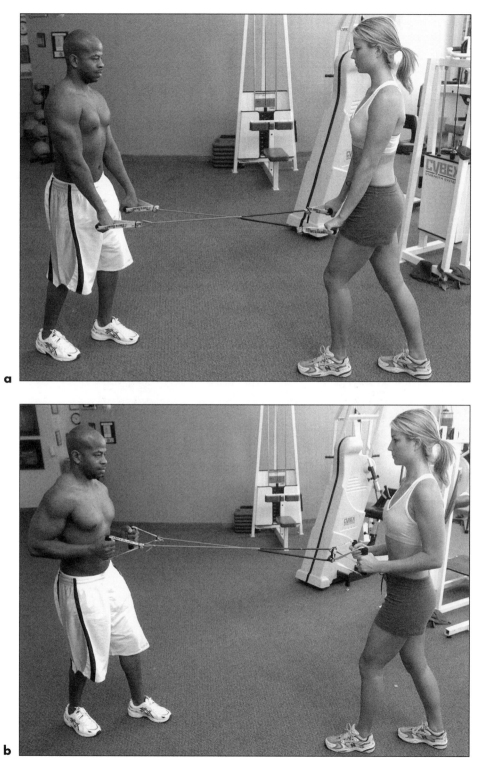

Figure 7.4 *(a)* Partner extension exercise, *(b)* partner pull.

Therarobics

Fitness and therapy experts from Europe developed a unique elastic-based fitness program called "Therarobics." The concept integrates whole-body exercise with one elastic device that connects the upper and lower extremities. By focusing on whole-body, multiple joint, and externally rotated movements, the Therarobics program has proven to be an excellent conditioning tool for many populations, including healthy adults and seniors. By using the Therarobics system, choreographed upper-body movements and lower-body movements are performed together to music. Therarobics combines strength, cardio, and balance training in one efficient system (see figures 7.5a-d).

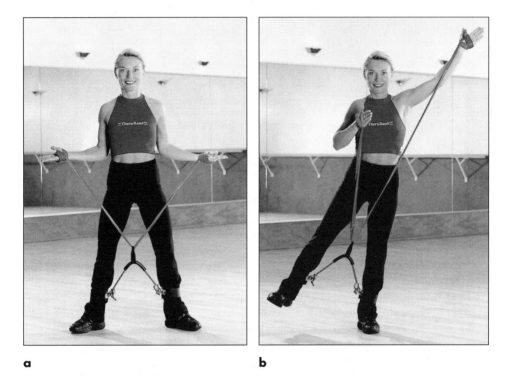

a   **b**

Figure 7.5   Sample Therarobics movements.

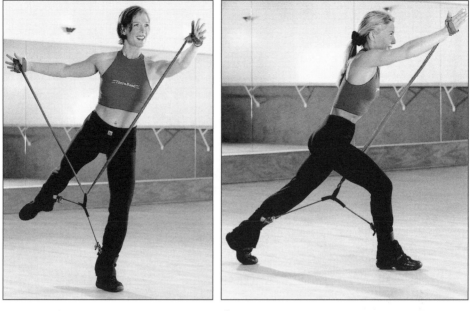

c   d

Aquatic Programs

Its physical properties make water an excellent setting for exercise. For example, the viscosity of water creates resistance to movement. In addition, the buoyancy decreases the stress on weight-bearing joints. This same buoyancy, however, prevents effective resistance training because it decreases the effect of gravity, therefore reducing the effectiveness of isotonic resistance exercises. In order to add resistance training to aquatic exercise routines, elastic resistance can be used in a pool to compensate for the reduced effects. Group aquatic programs for individuals with osteoarthritis and fibromyalgia are becoming more and more popular. Adding elastic resistance helps facilitate strengthening exercises in these populations as it takes the weight off of joints.

Caring for Elastic Bands in Aquatics . . . .

Follow these care guidelines for bands used in aquatic exercises.

- Rinse bands in clean, nonchlorinated water.
- Hang or lay flat to dry.
- Inspect bands for wear, and replace damaged bands.
- Use handles to avoid slippage.

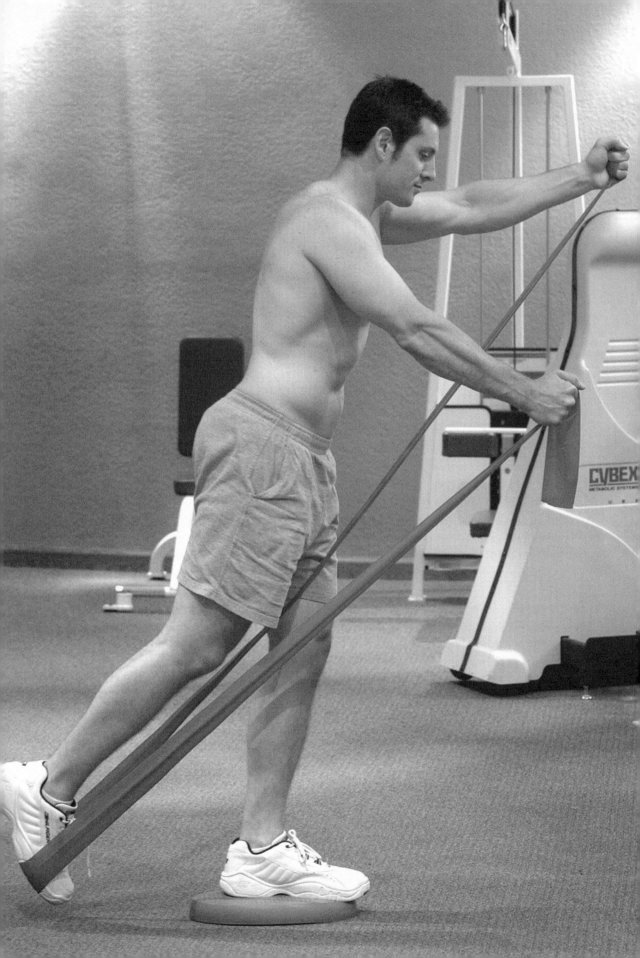

Chapter 8 ....

Power, Agility, and Speed Exercises

Elastic resistance can be used to improve power, agility, and speed. All general physical-fitness activities require some combination of these three abilities. One of the goals of sport-specific training is to incorporate these variables to optimize performance and prevent injury. For example, in a sport like tennis, which requires multidirectional movements performed explosively on a repetitive basis, training exercises that emphasize power, agility, and speed are necessary to help a player achieve full potential. An understanding of how elastic resistance can be used to improve these important aspects of performance can be gained by defining each of these parameters.

Power can be defined as the ability to exert or produce force in a very short period. Agility is the ability to accelerate, decelerate, and change directions quickly while keeping good body control. Finally, speed may be defined as the rate at which body segments move. Elastic resistance used to assist in shortening (concentric), lengthening (eccentric), and stabilizing (isometric) muscle work enhances the development of power, agility, and speed. There are several exercise applications where elastic bands and tubing can be used to improve speed, agility, and power. In addition to acceleration training, deceleration training, and overload, plyometrics is one of the most successful methods to improve speed and power.

• **Acceleration Training.** Several of the exercises in this chapter, such as throwing and assisted running and sprinting, utilize the concept of acceleration training. While there are many definitions that apply to this type of training, most simply, elastic resistance can be used to increase the speed that a body segment, or series of body segments, moves. For example, to increase running speed, a partner exercise can be used that stretches the elastic tubing to a point of tension so that as the exercising person begins to run, the taut band causes the runner to move at a faster rate than if unassisted. Assisted training is another term commonly used for this type of exercise. Elastic resistance exercise is ideal for this type of training because of the long distances used when training the lower body as well as the long lengths of material needed to perform this type of assisted training. The figures on page 125 show a shoulder exercise for throwing or overhead athletics, when the arm is accelerated forward into internal rotation using a prestretched length of elastic tubing.

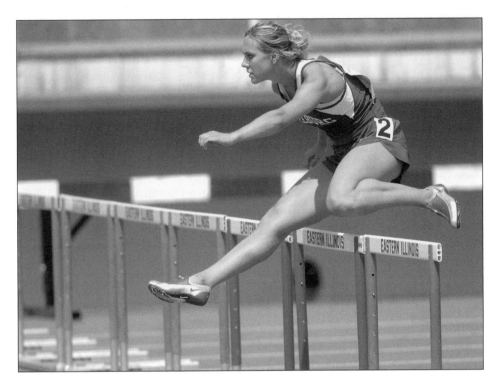

Speed and agility training can be incorporated into your elastic resistance progam.

• **Deceleration Training.** Another commonly used technique is to train the body during lengthening contractions or situations when the body is decelerating. An example of this type of training is the squat, when additional resistance is applied by prestretched elastic resistance during the descent phase of the squat to train the quadriceps muscle eccentrically (or during lengthening). This eccentric muscle work is extremely functional and has direct application in the lower body for activities such as landing from a jump and absorbing the load from the body during directional changes inherent in nearly all sports. Elastic resistance is again an excellent choice as a resistance medium as it has an inherent eccentric property. Once the band or tubing is stretched, the participant must work against the resistance that has been created eccentrically as the exercise movement continues to the starting position. Eccentric training is important not only in performance enhancement and injury prevention, but also rehabilitation programs. The inclusion of eccentrics in the training program addresses the need to control the body segments and provide stability.

• **Overload.** One of the most widely accepted theories in strength training is that an overload stress to the muscle is needed for muscular strength development to take place. Again, elastic resistance exercise can be used to provide the necessary overload. The figures on pages 126–129 show how elastic bands can be used to provide the overload to the lower extremity musculature during forward, backward, lateral, and carioca movements to train the muscles in an explosive manner with the appropriate level of overload. An optimal resistance level must be used to allow the body segments to move explosively and, at the same time, receive enough resistance for adaptation to occur. Too much resistance won't allow normal coordinated movements to occur at optimal velocities and will detract from the development of power and speed. Elastic resistance provides resistance along many lines of force, or vectors of resistance, that re-creates sport-specific movement patterns. For example, the figure on page 130 shows how elastic resistance can be used to resist a tennis player's movement along the baseline by resisting the appropriate movement vector simulating a movement that actually occurs during tennis.

• **Plyometrics.** Plyometric exercise contains three components: an eccentric or lengthening muscle contraction (phase one), immediately followed by a strong, forceful, rapid concentric contraction (phase two), and the amortization phase (phase three), consisting of the very short time between the lengthening contraction (eccentric) and the shortening contraction (concentric). The longer the amortization phase, the less optimal the plyometric exercise. In order for the plyometric contraction to be successful, the load and movement pattern used during the exercise must allow for a rapid stretch of the contracting musculature followed by a very short amortization phase to produce the optimal explosive shortening contraction. Elastic resistance can be used as an adjunct to traditional plyometric exercise by providing additional overload and also to provide additional resistance and stresses to the body during the performance of the exercise. The figures on page 131 show how a simple lateral step jump can be complemented with elastic resistance.

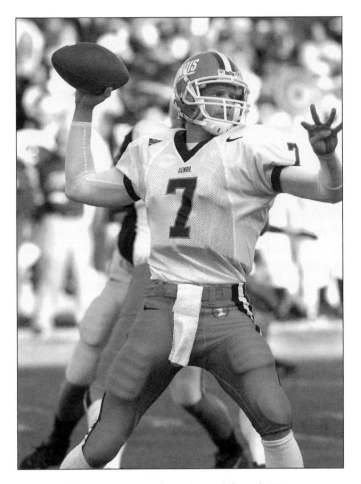

Sport-specific movements can be enhanced through ERT.

Another example of plyometrics using elastic resistance is pictured on page 132. This external rotation plyometric drill is a great exercise for overhead athletics such as baseball and tennis, and uses a position that simulates the throwing motion and tennis serve. The athlete uses a starting position of 90 degrees of external rotation and then forcefully internally rotates the shoulder to obtain a prestretch to the external rotator muscles in the back of the shoulder. After attaining the internal rotation position, the arm is immediately brought back to the starting position against the resistance of elastic tubing. This is an excellent example of how elastic resistance can be used in a safe and controlled manner to perform movement patterns at faster speeds for sport specificity. This exercise provides extremely important strength to the rotator cuff musculature and is highly recommended to promote muscle balance and rotator cuff strength in overhead athletics.

The following pages show additional exercises using elastic resistance to improve power, agility, and speed.

ASSISTED THROWING

Secure tubing at shoulder height and stand sideways (throwing arm farthest away) to the attachment holding the tubing in the throwing hand. Assume cocking position of the throwing motion and stand at a distance so a moderate amount of resistance is placed on tubing (a). Quickly accelerate arm forward using normal throwing motion (b). The tension in tubing is used to overaccelerate arm to build arm speed.

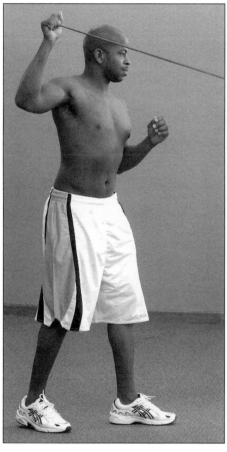
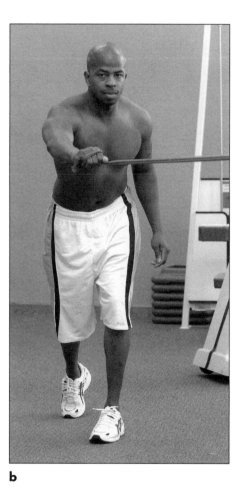

a   **b**

RESISTED FORWARD RUNNING

Stand with band or tubing wrapped around waist and partner holding other ends from behind, but far enough away not to interfere with running *(a)*. Begin running forward against resistance of elastic tubing and partner *(b)*.

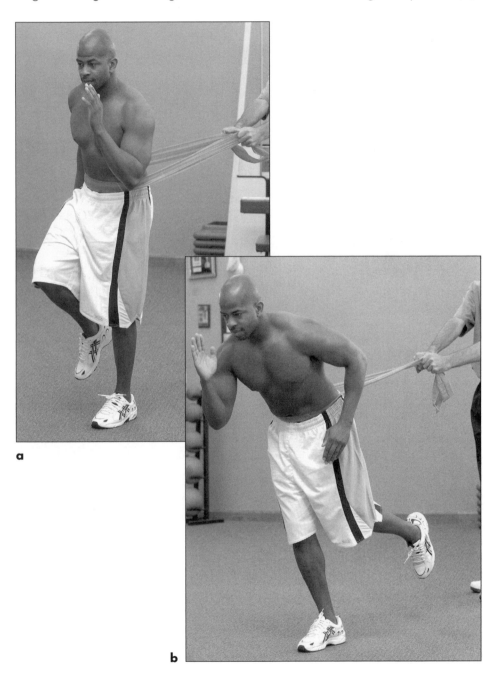

a

b

RESISTED BACKWARD RUNNING

Stand with band or tubing secured around waist and a partner holding other end from front, but far enough away not to interfere with running (a). Begin running backward against elastic resistance and partner (b).

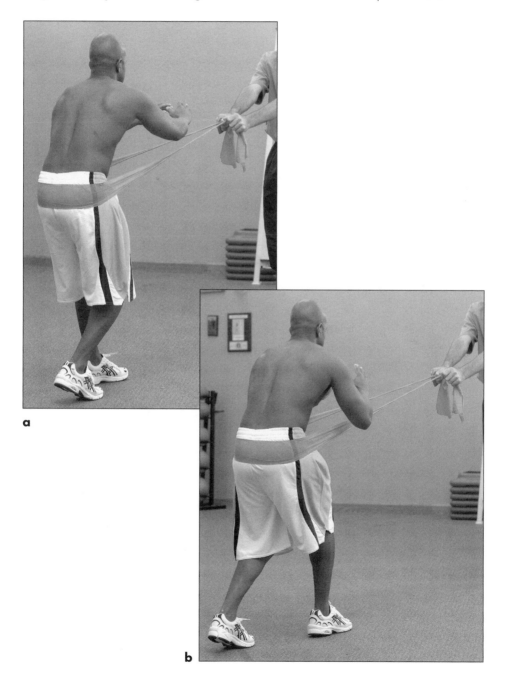

a

b

RESISTED LATERAL RUNNING

Stand with band or tubing secured around waist and partner holding other end from side, but far enough away not to interfere with running *(a)*. Begin running, or shuffling, sideways against resistance and partner *(b)*. Switch directions for balanced training.

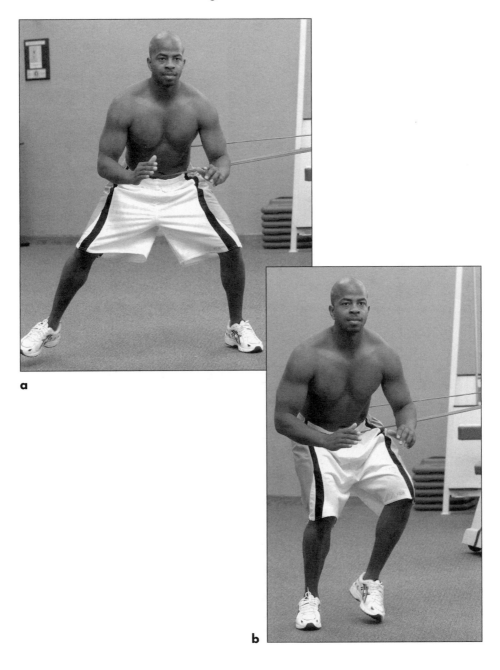

a

b

RESISTED CARIOCA

Stand with band or tubing secured around waist and partner holding other end from side, but far enough away not to interfere with running *(a)*. Begin moving sideways, alternating steps in front of and behind the other leg, (carioca steps) against elastic resistance and partner *(b)*.

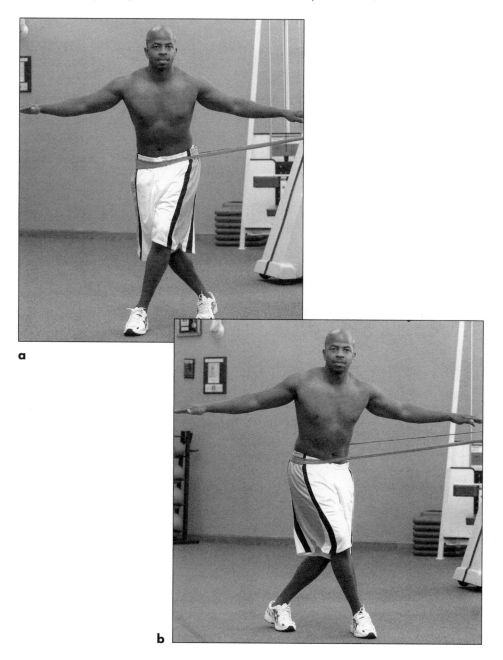

a

b

RESISTED LATERAL MOVEMENT

Stand on baseline of tennis court in ready position with racket in hand. Secure band or tubing around waist with partner holding other ends from side, but far enough away not to interfere with movement (a). Simulate a backhand groundstroke to begin lateral motion. Complete 1-2 steps to finalize stroke position against resistance (b). Repeat on forehand side by having partner stand on opposite side.

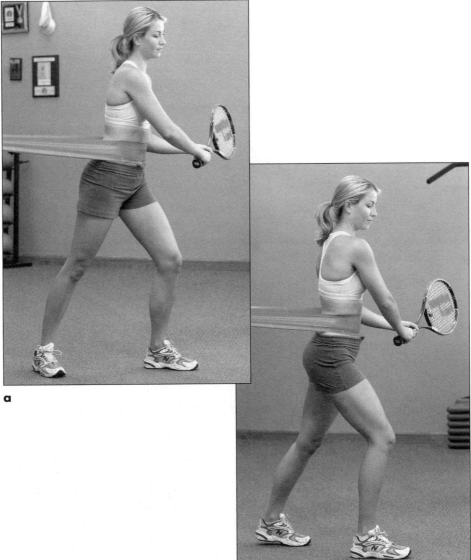

a

b

RESISTED LATERAL JUMP STEP PLYOMETRIC

Stand with one foot on top of step platform. Secure band or tubing around waist with other ends held by partner or secured at waist height to stationary object (a). Jump across step away from attachment, placing foot on top with each crossing (b). Alternate feet placed on top of step. Tubing provides resistance during jump away from attachment and assistance toward attachment.

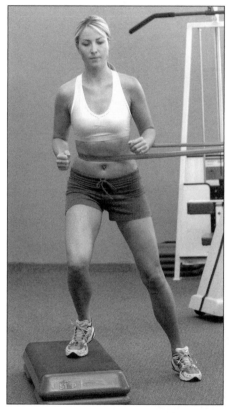

a

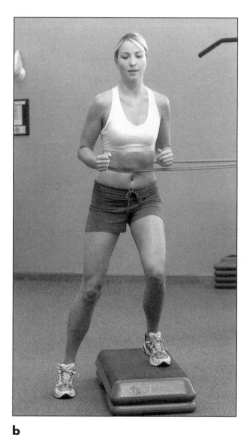

b

EXTERNAL ROTATION PLYOMETRIC 90/90 POSITION

Secure band or tubing at shoulder level and stand facing attachment with shoulder elevated to 90 degrees. The arm should be slightly (about 30 degrees) in front of body as pictured, not directly to side *(a)*. Start with forearm in vertical position with moderate tension on tubing. Begin by quickly moving shoulder until forearm becomes horizontal *(b)*, and then without pausing, move arm back to starting position. While movement of arm is most noticeable, shoulder rotation is being trained on this exercise. Additionally, elbow and shoulder remain bent at 90 degrees.

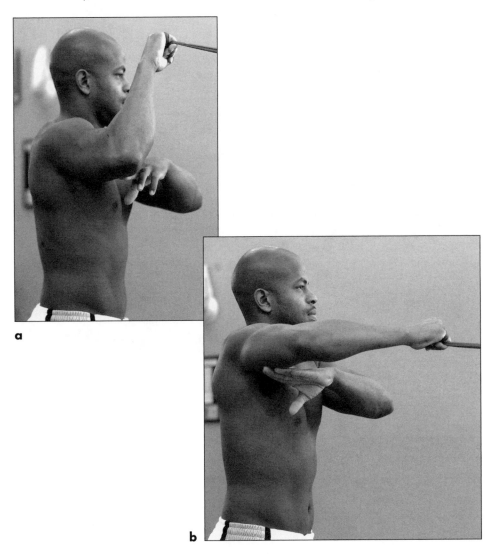

a

b

SQUAT WITH ELASTIC BAND ON BARBELL

Start in squat position. Several variations can be used, such as front squat. Secure two pieces of band or tubing, one on each end of barbell, to a sturdy object on floor or under your feet *(a)*. Secure tubing so that moderate resistance is present when squat exercise is in ascent phase. Perform squat exercise using normal form with the additional resistance from band or tubing *(b)*.

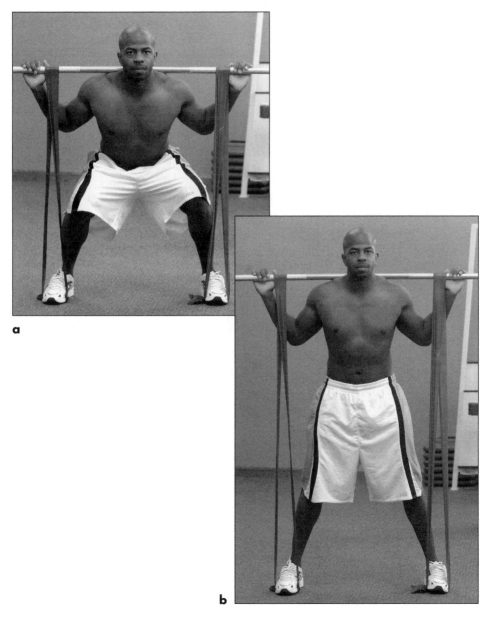

a

b

DEADLIFT WITH ELASTIC BAND ON BARBELL

Secure two pieces of elastic band or tubing on each end of barbell and other end to floor. Stand with feet shoulder-width apart. Squat next to bar with arms outside knees *(a)*. With back straight and shoulders directly over or slightly in front of bar, extend knees and move hips forward, lifting bar upward *(b)*. Bands provide additional resistance to movement. Slowly return barbell to floor.

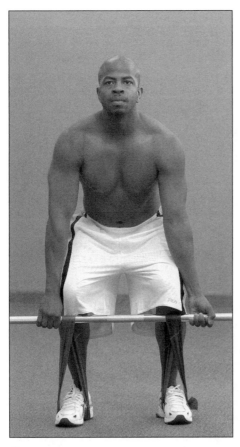

a

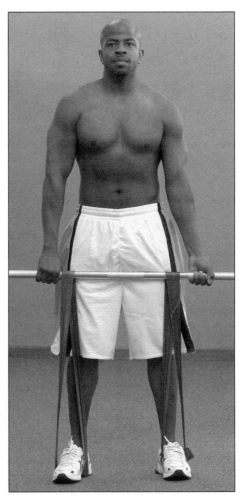

b

ARM ACCELERATION DRILL (PNF D2 Diagonal)

Secure tubing at knee level and face attachment. Grab other end of band or tubing in starting position with arm overhead with thumb pointing backward (a). Stand at distance from attachment so moderate resistance is present. Move arm forward in diagonal pattern similar to throwing motion with the band (b), and work against the resistance of the band moving back to starting position.

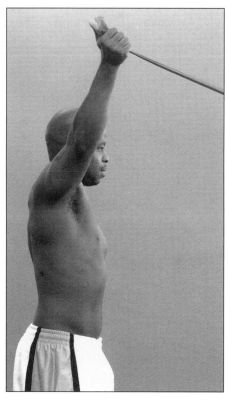

a

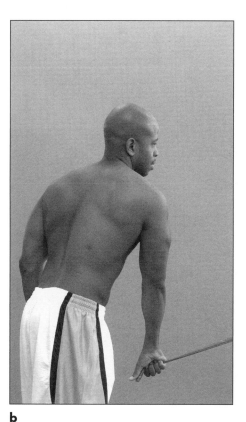

b

STEP JUMP WITH ELASTIC RESISTANCE

Stand with elastic band or tubing around waist, the other end held either by partner or secured at waist height from behind. Place step platform in front, and jump up off step, alternating feet and keeping body posture erect and well balanced against resistance.

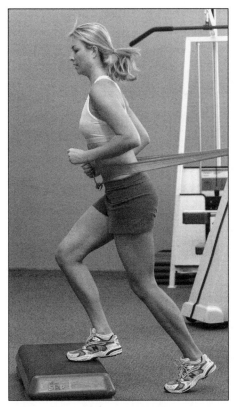

a

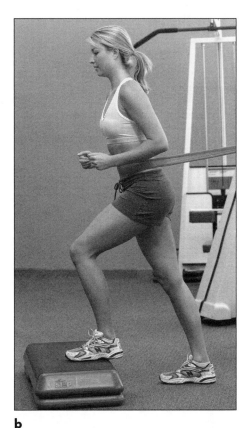

b

ASSISTED SPRINTING

Stand with elastic band or tubing around waist, the other end held by partner in front, but far enough away not to interfere with several steps of explosive forward movement (a). Elastic resistance should have moderate tension. Sprint several steps with assistance from the band propelling each step forward (b). The exercise ends when tension in band becomes insignificant.

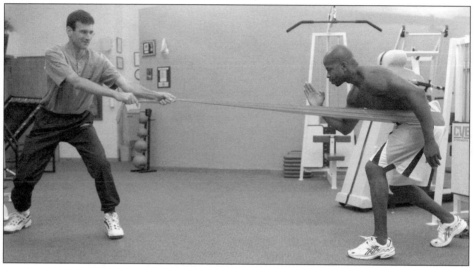

a

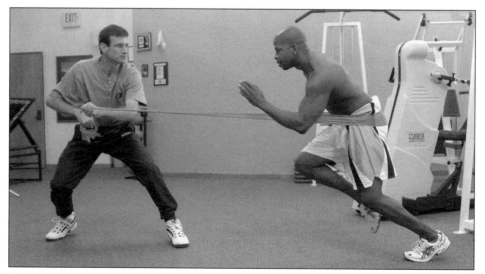

b

LATERAL BOUNDING

Stand with elastic band or tubing around waist, the other end held by a partner, but far enough away not to interfere with the movements needed to perform lateral bounding (a). Elastic resistance should have moderate tension. Perform several repetitions of lateral bounding against resistance, emphasizing high knees (b).

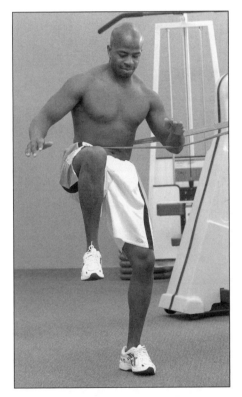

a

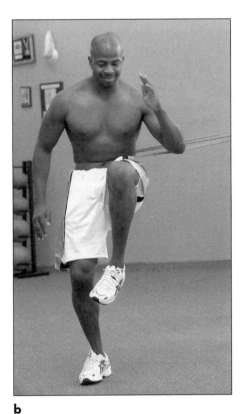

b

RESISTED STEP-UP AND STEP-OVER

Stand in front of step platform with band or tubing secured around waist, the other end held by partner from behind or secured to stationary object. Set band with enough tension to step up and over platform *(a)*, touching foot down on other side of platform *(b)*. Reverse to the starting position. Perform movement in controlled fashion. Repeat using other leg.

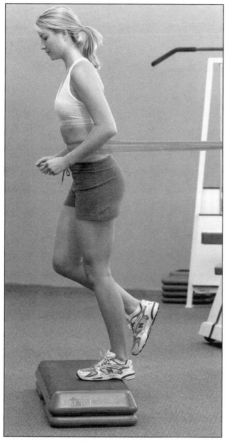

a

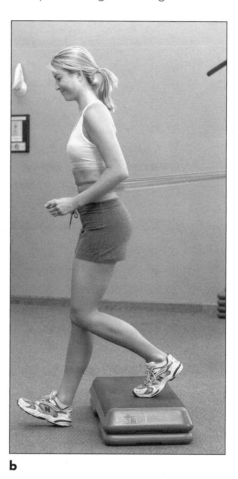

b

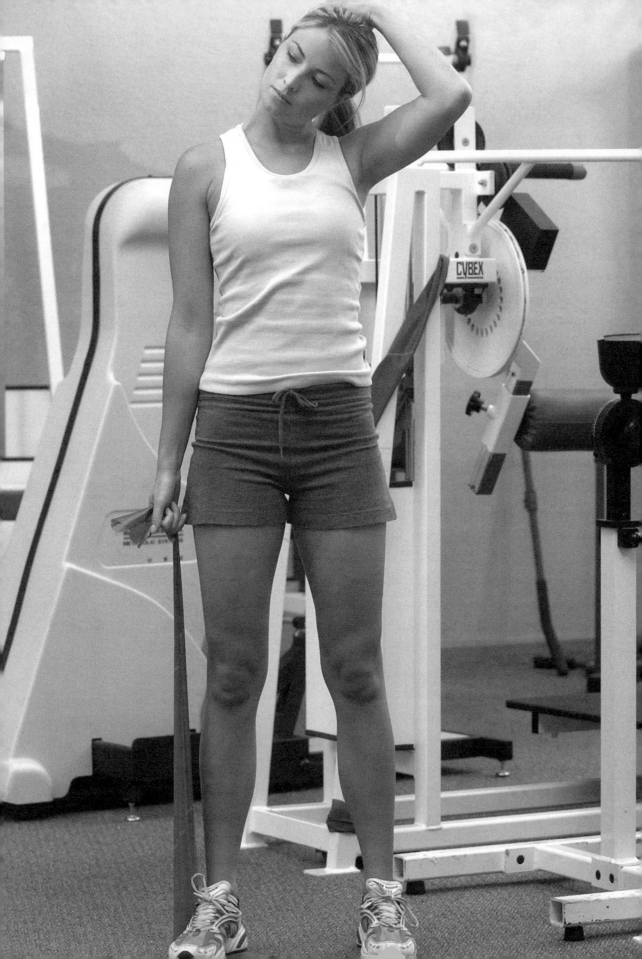

Chapter 9.............................
Stretching Exercises

Elastic resistance can be used to assist with stretching programs. Performing a contraction of the muscle before stretching makes the stretch more effective. This technique is known as pre-contraction stretch, when the muscle is contracted against the resistance of the band followed by a slow stretch to increase the length of the muscle. Research has shown that a prestretch contraction is a more effective way to increase muscle length and joint range of motion than a static stretch. For example, contracting the hamstrings against resistance prior to stretching will result in more range of motion at the hip. A prestretch contraction helps relax neurologically, and also increases the temperature of the muscle, making it more pliable and easier to stretch.

Several variations of precontraction stretching are based on proprioceptive neuromuscular facilitation (PNF) techniques, such as hold-relax and contract-relax. The most popular type, hold-relax stretching, involves taking the joint to the end range of motion, maximally elongating the muscle to be stretched. The muscle is then contracted with no joint movement, or isometrically, for approximately five seconds. Take up the slack at end range, holding the new stretch position between 10 and 30 seconds. Repeat this technique three or four times. Similarly, contract-relax stretching involves moving the joint through its entire range of motion (contracting the muscle to be stretched through its movement pattern) before returning to the end stretch position.

When choosing the resistance level of the band, use a high resistance that provides a comfortable stretch, but allows the muscle to isometrically contract (hold–relax) or the joint to move through the range of motion (contract–relax). Finally, remember to breathe normally, and don't hold your breath while stretching.

UPPER TRAPEZIUS

Stand on middle of band with one foot. Grasp one end of band and stretch band with hand of side being stretched. With other hand, grasp side of head and look down and away from side being stretched. Keeping elbow straight, shrug shoulder upward, pulling band toward ceiling, and inhale. Hold two to six seconds, then slowly allow band to return shoulder to starting position on the exhale. Hold stretch on band an additional 10 to 30 seconds. Repeat 3-4 times.

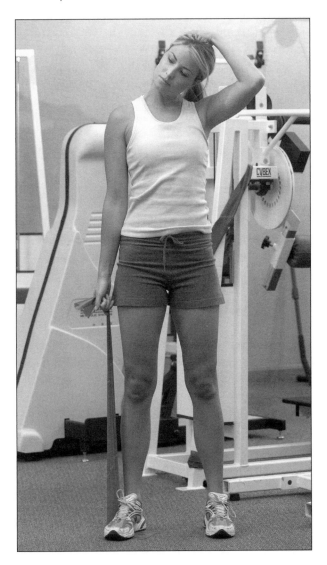

PECTORALIS MAJOR

Secure ends of looped band behind you at shoulder level. Stand with shoulder and elbow bent 90 degrees. Grasp middle of loop and allow band to stretch front part of shoulder. Keeping elbow bent, gently rotate shoulder inward against band, and inhale. Hold two to six seconds, then slowly allow band to return shoulder to starting position on the exhale. Hold stretch on band an additional 10 to 30 seconds. Repeat 3-4 times.

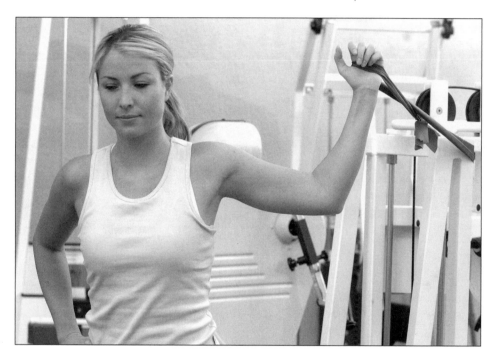

QUADRICEPS AND RECTUS FEMORIS

Lie on stomach with middle of band looped around shin. Secure ends of looped band in your hands. Gently extend knee, stretching band, and inhale. Hold two to six seconds, then slowly allow band to return leg to starting position on the exhale. Hold stretch on band an additional 10 to 30 seconds. Repeat 3-4 times.

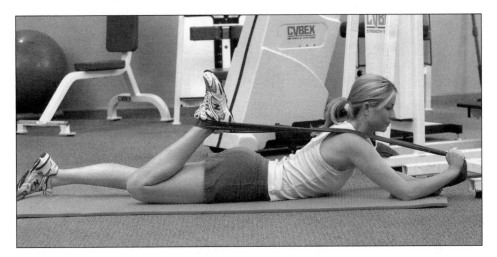

ILIOTIBIAL BAND

Secure ends of looped band to bedpost or table leg. Lie on side with leg being stretched hanging over table or bed. Flex hip on opposite leg. Wrap looped band around thigh and gently lift leg, stretching band, and inhale. Hold two to six seconds, then slowly allow band to return leg to starting position on the exhale. Hold stretch on band an additional 10 to 30 seconds. Repeat 3-4 times.

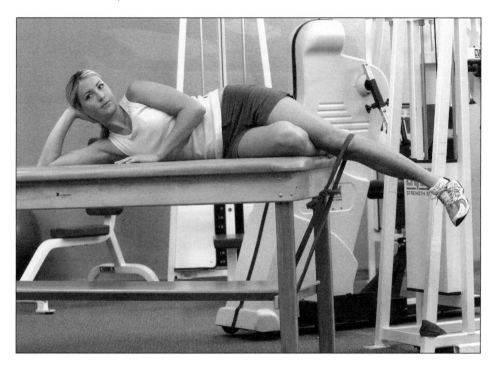

HIP FLEXORS AND ILIOPSOAS

Secure ends of looped band to bedpost or table leg. Lie on back with leg hanging over table or bed. Wrap looped band around the thigh and gently flex hip upward against the taut band, and inhale. Hold two to six seconds, then slowly allow band to return leg to starting position on the exhale. Hold stretch on band an additional 10 to 30 seconds. Repeat 3-4 times.

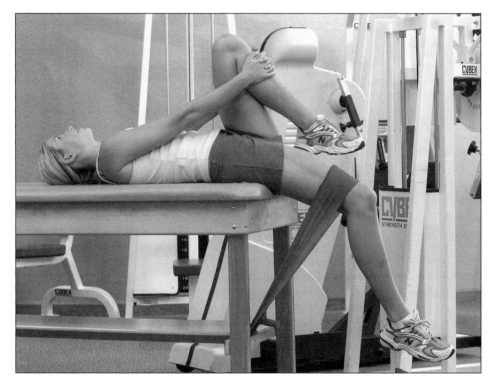

PIRIFORMIS

Lie on back with knee of side being stretched bent across opposite knee. Loop band around top knee, and grasp ends of band with hand on opposite side being stretched. Keep band taut and gently push top knee into band, and inhale. Hold two to six seconds, then slowly allow band to return leg to starting position on the exhale. Hold stretch on band an additional 10 to 30 seconds. Repeat 3-4 times.

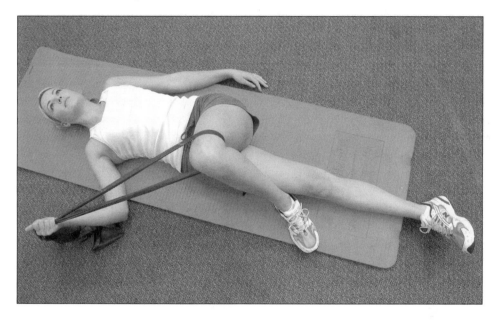

HAMSTRINGS

Lie on back with looped band around foot or ankle of the leg being stretched. Lift extended leg, and grasp ends of band, pulling leg upward. Gently push extended leg downward against band, keeping knee straight. Hold two to six seconds, then slowly allow band to return leg to starting position on the exhale. Hold stretch on band an additional 10 to 30 seconds. Repeat 3-4 times.

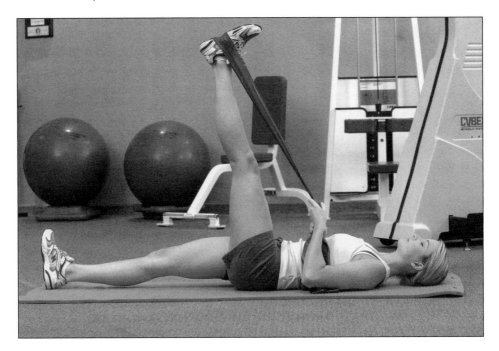

GASTROCNEMIUS AND SOLEUS

Sit with knees extended with looped band around foot being stretched. Grasp ends of band, pulling foot backward. Gently push foot downward against band, keeping knee straight. Hold two to six seconds, then slowly allow band to return leg to starting position on the exhale. Hold stretch on band an additional 10 to 30 seconds. Repeat 3-4 times. To isolate the soleus, perform same stretch with knee slightly bent instead of straight (pictured).

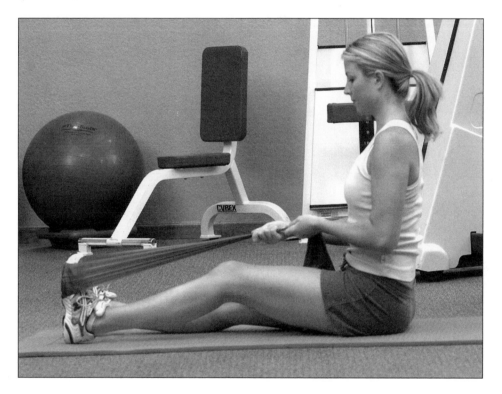

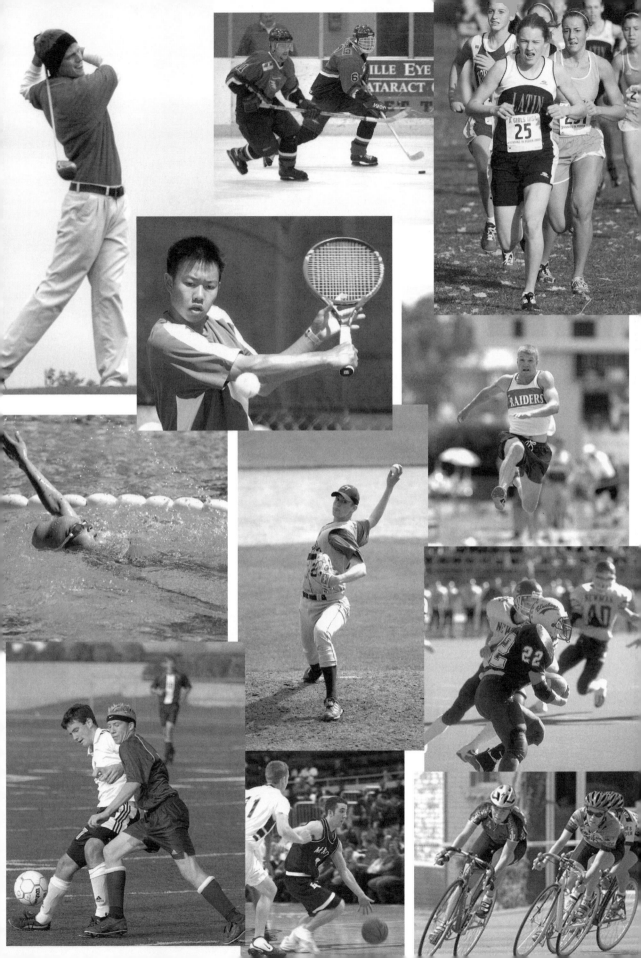

Chapter 10..........................
Functional Training Programs

The limitless applications and exercises possible with elastic resistance make it ideal for athletes seeking to perform sport-specific training. Additionally, the fact that elastic resistance is portable makes it ideal for the athlete to train while traveling (chapter 11), or on the courts and athletic fields. The purpose of this chapter will be to briefly describe some of the specific physical demands of a sport, followed by specific exercises that serve both to prevent injury in that sport as well as enhance performance. Because repetitive performance in most sports often leads to an imbalance in muscular development, injury can result. In many cases, elastic resistance exercise can be used to improve balance of opposing muscle forces. Exercises in this chapter are listed after each sport. The exercises are divided into two groups: Base exercises are essential to the sport for balancing muscle

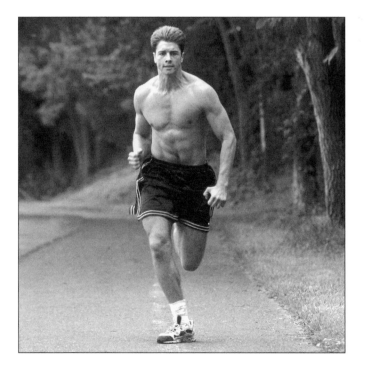

Using ERT to maintain balance in muscular development will help to prevent injuries.

groups as well as improving strength and endurance of key muscles; sport specific exercises simulate movement patterns inherent in that activity. Performing a combination of base exercises and sport specific exercises is recommended.

Baseball and Softball

The demands of baseball and softball encompass all areas of the body but particularly stress the shoulder and elbow. Injuries from inadequate strength and muscle endurance of the rotator cuff and scapular stabilizers (muscles that stabilize the shoulder blade, such as the rhomboids, trapezius, and serratus anterior) are common. Additionally, strong forceful trunk rotation is needed for both throwing and batting, making core stability an essential part of any baseball or softball conditioning program. Finally, explosive lower-body propulsive movements are important in nearly all positions and in base running.

BASE EXERCISES
Shoulder external rotation at 90 degrees (page 20)

Wrist flexion and extension (page 30)

Supination and pronation (page 32)

Seated row (page 38)

Squat (page 96)

Lunge (page 98)

Standing extension with retraction (page 153)

Linton external rotation (page 154)

SPORT SIMULATION EXERCISES
Batting simulation two-hand rotation (page 155)

Lateral step with glove (page 156)

Throwing simulation (page 157)

STANDING EXTENSION WITH RETRACTION (THUMB OUT) (Latissimus Dorsi, Posterior Deltoid, Teres Major)

Secure middle of band or tubing at chest level to stationary object. Face attachment and grasp ends. Flex arms with thumb pointing outward (supinated forearm position). Slowly move arm backward toward side, keeping elbow straight . Slowly return. Repeat.

Training Tip

As arm moves backward, squeeze shoulder blades together to activate rhomboids and trapezius muscles.

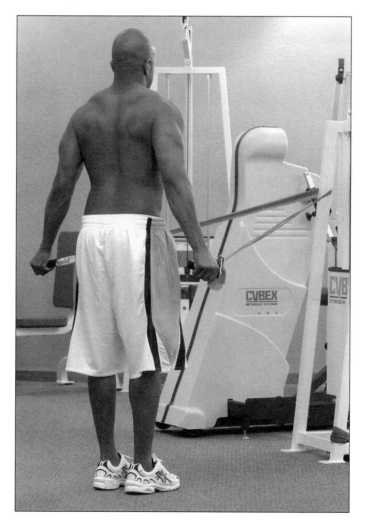

LINTON EXTERNAL ROTATION (Rotator Cuff, Rhomboids, Trapezius, Posterior Deltoids)

Kneel, securing elastic band or tubing under opposite hand with the other end held in the hand of the shoulder your are training. Keep elbow bent and arm across abdomen. Keep head and spine in neutral position. Externally rotate shoulder (as pictured) and extend arm upward straightening elbow. Slowly return.

Training Tip

As arm extends upward, squeeze shoulder blades together to increase the work on rhomboids and trapezius muscles.

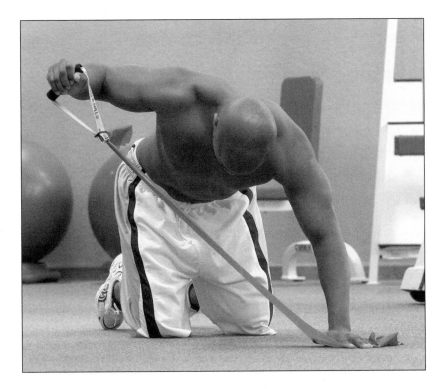

BATTING SIMULATION TWO-HAND ROTATION
(Trunk Rotators, Gluteals, Quadriceps, Calves)

Secure band or tubing to bat handle and assume batting stance. Simulate swing to point just beyond normal contact of ball.

Training Tip

Attach tubing to different points along bat to vary resistance to certain muscle groups. The farther tubing is anchored from hands the greater wrist and forearm activity.

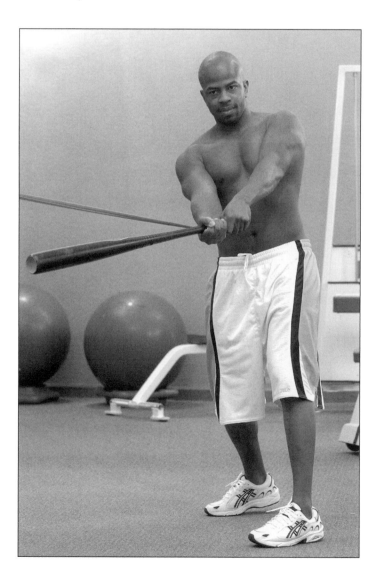

LATERAL STEP WITH GLOVE (All Muscle Groups)

Simulates fielding with lateral movement. Secure ends of band or have partner hold ends of elastic band. Wrap middle of band around waist, and take large controlled step away from attachment, and bend to simulate fielding a ball.

Training Tip

Use different directions of resistance. For example, resisting on a diagonal and going forward and to one side simulates moving in to field a ball.

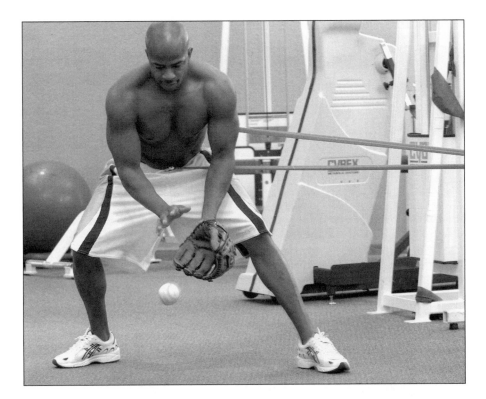

THROWING SIMULATION (All Muscle Groups)

Grasp one end of band or tubing and secure the other end of the tubing at shoulder level in a door or on a secure object such as a fence. Face away from attachment and perform a throwing motion, including follow-through, using resistance from band to gently overload the muscles used in throwing.

Training Tip

This exercise is an ideal warm-up before throwing with very light bands as a form of dynamic warm-up.

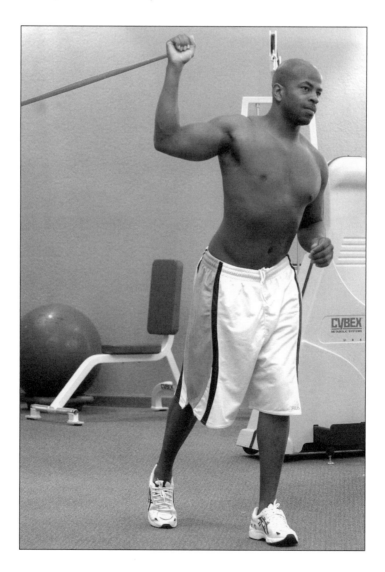

Football

Injuries and demands in football can range from overuse such as tendinitis and muscle strains to severe ligament injuries and even fractures. Football is classified not as a contact sport but a collision sport with a wide range of injury and performance patterns based on field position. The ability to move in multiple directions and have explosive upper-extremity power is essential in nearly all positions. In addition, multiple-joint and whole-body movements are often more important to strengthen multiple muscles rather than exercises that isolate joints and work primarily one muscle group.

BASE EXERCISES
Bench press (page 36)

Squat (page 96)

Lunge (page 98)

Monster walk (page 159)

SPORT SIMULATION EXERCISES
Resisted backward running (page 127)

Explosion out of three-point stance (page 160)

Total-body extension (page 161)

Rip (page 162)

MONSTER WALK (Hip Abductors, Core)

Loop band around lower legs just inches above ankles. Stand with slight bend in hips and knees in a "ready" position. Take wide step to one side then the other against resistance of band. Continue moving in a shuffling motion, taking multiple steps.

Training Tip

Use multiple directions including sideways and diagonal, as well as front and back.

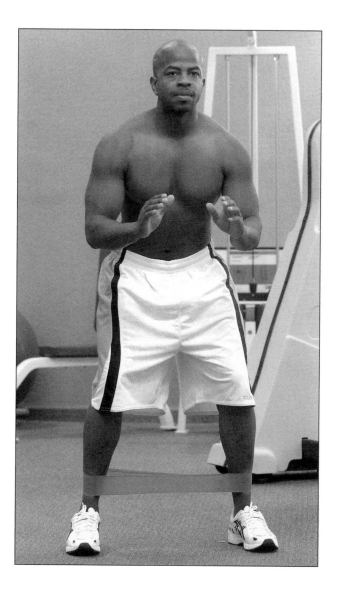

EXPLOSION OUT OF THREE-POINT STANCE
(All Muscle Groups)

Start in three-point stance with middle of band or tubing secured around waist and partner holding other end. Player explodes out of stance and takes one step forward.

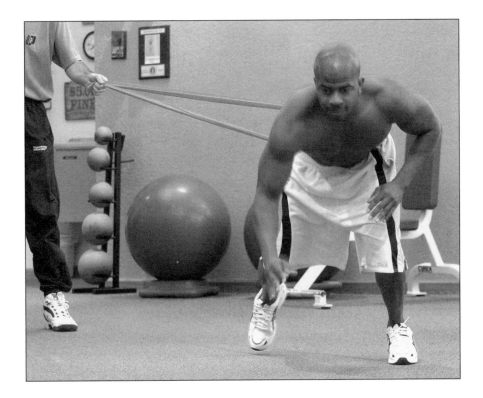

TOTAL-BODY EXTENSION (All Muscle Groups)

Loop band around backs of thighs. Grasp ends at shoulder level. Bend hips and knees, and assume crouch starting position. Extend arms forward and move out of crouch with lower body.

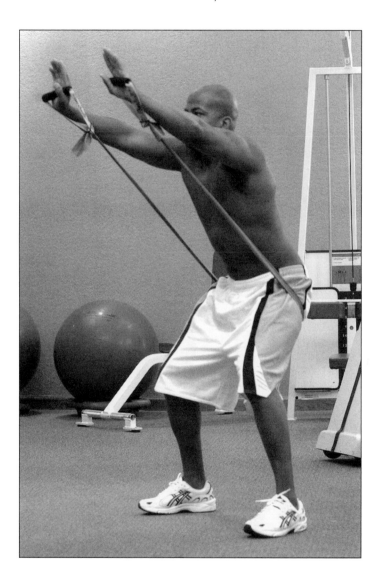

RIP (All Muscle Groups)

Secure band or tubing at shoulder level to stationary object behind you. Step forward with the opposite leg as the arm being resisted and move the arm across the body in a "rip" type motion. Perform with one arm, and then the other. This simulates upper-body movement for defensive linemen.

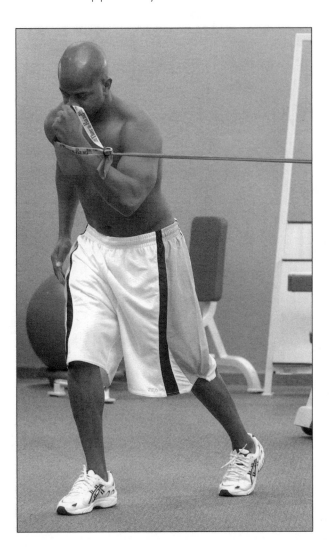

Soccer

The multidirectional movements and cutting patterns required in soccer produce large demands on the lower body. Additionally, strength and balance of the stance leg are essential for successful motion by the kicking leg. Hip flexibility and strength in relatively large ranges of motion involve muscles that cross both the hip and knee (including the groin, hamstrings, and quadriceps). Hip stretching and strengthening exercises are essential and should be emphasized. Functional diagonal movements of the lower body during kicking can also be performed against elastic resistance.

BASE EXERCISES

Dorsiflexion (page 102)

Plantar flexion (page 104)

Ankle inversion (page 106)

Ankle eversion (page 108)

Monster walk (page 159)

Closed-chain hip rotation (page 164)

SPORT SIMULATION EXERCISES

Abduction pattern with soccer ball (page 165)

Basic kicking diagonal (page 166)

Reciprocal arm and leg (page 167)

Concentric and eccentric hamstrings (page 168)

Throw-in simulation and overhead pass (page 169)

CLOSED-CHAIN HIP ROTATION (Hip Rotators)

Stand sideways to secure ends of band at knee-level and loop middle of band around ankle on the same side as hip to be exercised. Stand with exercising leg on exercise ball or chair. Rotate hip inward and outward against the resistance while stabilizing knee against ball. Turn body to face opposite direction to work the other direction of hip rotation.

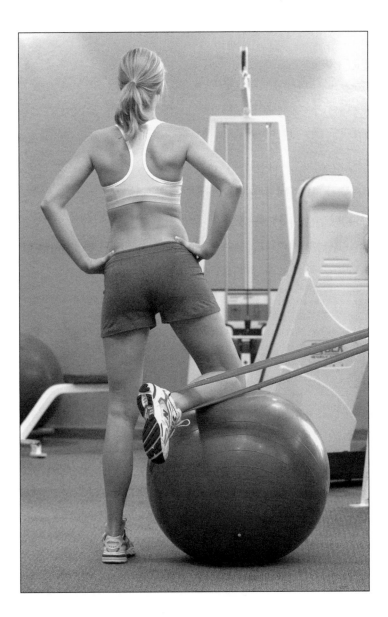

ABDUCTION PATTERN WITH SOCCER BALL
(Hip Abductors and Flexors)

Loop band or tubing around both ankles, or use an extremity strap to secure tubing to both ankles (pictured). Place soccer ball just in front and to side of starting position. Lunge forward toward the ball.

Training Tip

Repeat in multiple positions by changing position of ball.

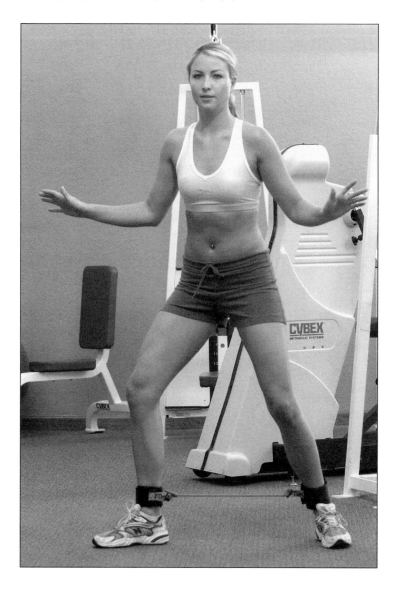

BASIC KICKING DIAGONAL
(All Muscle Groups)

Wrap one end of band around kicking leg near the ankle, and secure other end at waist level on a diagonal to a secure object behind you. Face away from attachment. Start with leg lifted behind with light tension on band. Simulate the kicking motion. Slowly return.

Training Tip

Stand on a foam surface with stance leg to increase difficulty and improve balance.

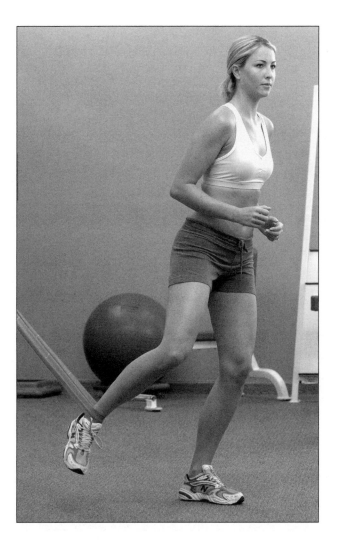

RECIPROCAL ARM AND LEG
(All Muscle Groups)

Secure band to stationary object at about knee level. Face away from attachment and loop middle of band around thigh. Flex leg forward (right leg), while pulling right arm backward and punching left arm forward. Slowly return. Repeat on opposite side.

Training Tip

Stand on a foam surface with stance leg to increase difficulty and improve balance.

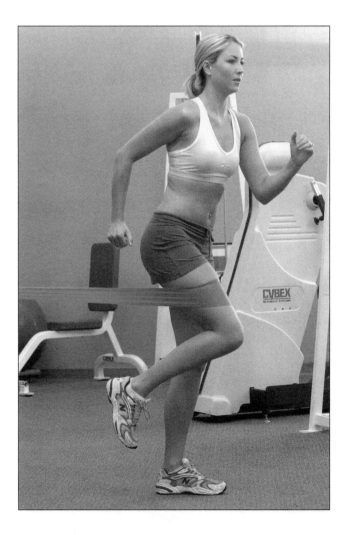

CONCENTRIC AND ECCENTRIC HAMSTRINGS (Gluteals, Hamstrings)

Stand on one leg with one end of the band secured at approximately waist level in a door or secure object. Wrap the other end of the band around your non-weightbearing leg just above the ankle. Maintain a secure balanced posture as pictured. Slowly bend the knee to approximately 90-100 degrees against the resistance, then slowly return to the starting position. Repeat.

Training Tip

Stand on a foam surface for more challenge.

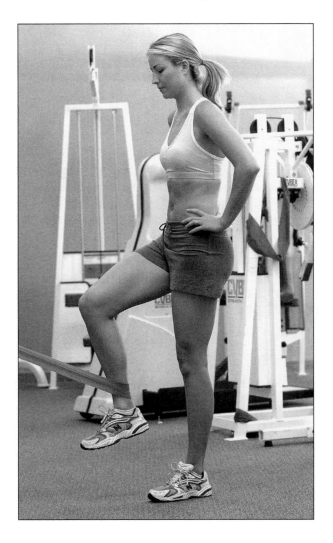

THROW-IN SIMULATION AND OVERHEAD PASS (Abdominals, Hip Flexors, Latissimus Dorsi)

Stand with arms overhead. Grasp middle of band or tubing with both hands. Secure other end of the tubing to stationary object at about eye level. Face away from attachment. Simulate soccer throw-in pattern, bending slightly forward at hips and trunk.

Training Tip
Combine with a twisting motion to train obliques.

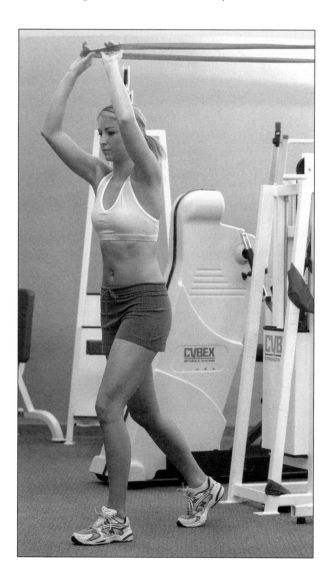

Tennis

The unique demands of tennis include multidirectional lower-body movement, aggressive trunk rotation, and very large concentric and eccentric stresses to the rotator cuff and scapular (shoulder blade) muscles. Additionally, research demonstrates high levels of muscle activity in the wrist and forearm during ground strokes and serving. It's important to train these muscles to prevent elbow and wrist injury. Tennis players demonstrate significantly greater shoulder and arm strength on the dominant racket arm; therefore, particular emphasis on the rotator cuff and upper-back muscles is also recommended.

BASE EXERCISES

Shoulder internal and external rotation (page 20)

Wrist flexion and extension (page 30)

Supination and pronation (page 32)

Monster walk (page 159). Add tennis racket to make exercise sport specific.

Wrist radial deviation (page 171)

Wrist ulnar deviation (page 172)

Unilateral row with side bridge (page 173)

Serratus punch (page 174)

SPORT SIMULATION EXERCISES

Open stance forehand resisted movement with racket (page 175)

Elbow extension with shoulder abduction (page 176)

Seated ball rotation with racket (page 177)

Horizontal abduction (page 178)

WRIST RADIAL DEVIATION

Begin in seated or standing position with the tubing held in the hand and secure the other end under the foot securely. If seated, rest the exercising arm on top of the thigh with the forearm in a neutral position such that the thumb is pointing directly upward (thumb up position). Beginning with the wrist bent downward toward the floor, and without moving the forearm away from its resting position on the thigh, bend the wrist in an upward direction as pictured. This is radial deviation. Slowly return to the starting position and repeat.

Training Tip

Use the opposite hand to stabilize the forearm position and ensure that it remains on the thigh throughout the exercise movement.

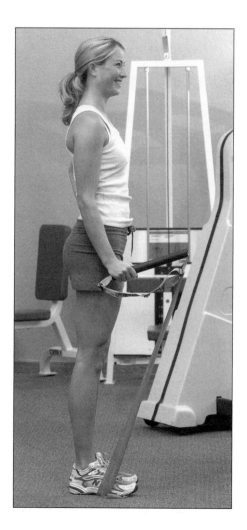

WRIST ULNAR DEVIATION

Begin in seated or standing position with the tubing held in the exercising hand and the other end of the tubing held in the other hand held approximately 6 inches directly above the exercising hand. Rest the exercising arm on top of the thigh with the forearm in a neutral position such that the thumb is pointing directly upward (thumb up position). Beginning with the wrist bent upward toward the ceiling, and without moving the forearm away from its resting position on the thigh, bend the wrist in a downward direction, as pictured. This is ulnar deviation. Slowly return to the starting position and repeat.

Training Tip

The movements of radial and ulnar deviation are not large, therefore don't force the motion. Work through the relatively short available movement pattern.

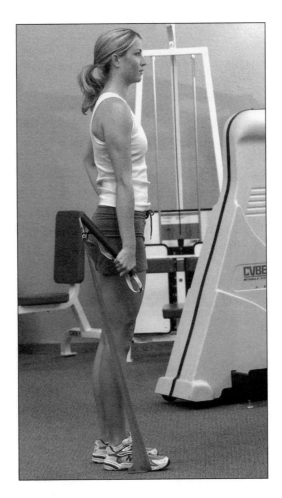

UNILATERAL ROW WITH SIDE BRIDGE (Core)

Lie on side, resting on elbow directly under shoulder. Keep body in alignment, tensing abdominal muscles and gluteal muscles. Use other hand to grasp tubing and perform one arm rowing exercise while stabilizing side bridge position.

Training Tip

Do exercise for both sides of body, not just rowing for your racket arm.

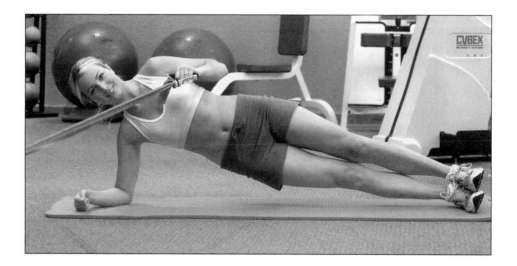

SERRATUS PUNCH (Serratus Anterior)

Secure tubing on stationary object at shoulder level. Face away from attachment and grasp end. Keeping elbow straight, punch forward, moving shoulder blade forward. Note: This involves a small, 6-inch movement. Slowly return.

Training Tip
Avoid rotating trunk to best isolate the serratus anterior muscle.

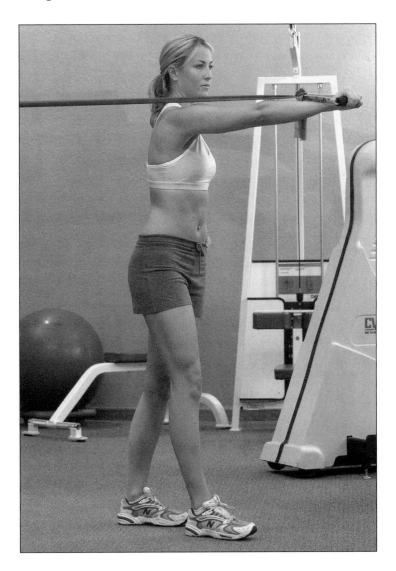

OPEN STANCE FOREHAND RESISTED MOVEMENT WITH RACKET (All Muscle Groups)

Wrap middle of band around waist and stand in ready position with ends secured at waist-level, or with partner holding other end of band. Step laterally using an open stance while simulating a forehand with racket in hand. Slowly return. Repeat.

Training Tip

Slowly control motion back to starting position to work muscles.

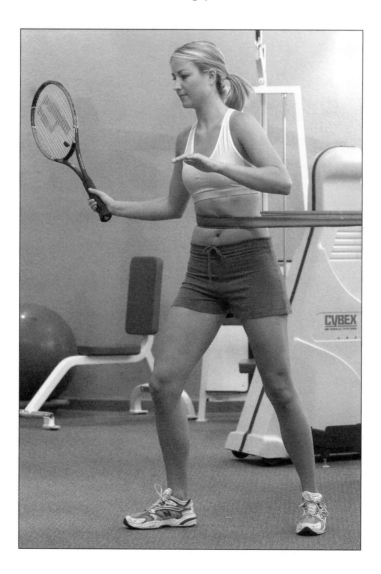

ELBOW EXTENSION WITH SHOULDER ABDUCTION (SERVE SIMULATION) (Triceps)

Stand with band or tubing under one foot and shoulder at about 100 degrees and elbow bent 90 degrees. Lean to the side with trunk approximately 30 degrees to simulate the serving position, and extend elbow. Slowly return elbow to starting position and repeat.

Training Tip

Stabilize arm using other hand to ensure that shoulder stays in serving position. Note: Avoid placing shoulder in overhead position because during serve the shoulder is elevated only 90 to 100 degrees due to side bend of trunk.

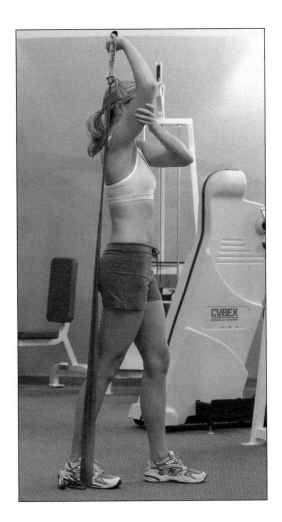

SEATED BALL ROTATION WITH RACKET
(Obliques, Core)

Secure one end of band or tubing to an attachment next to you and grasp other end of band. Sit on exercise ball and hold tennis racket with both hands straight out in front. Sit tall and tense abdominal muscles. Rotate to one side, keeping elbows extended. Slowly return to starting position.

Training Tip

Rotate to both sides by facing other direction. Keep feet on floor. It is important to perform rotation to both sides. To do this, simply face the other direction.

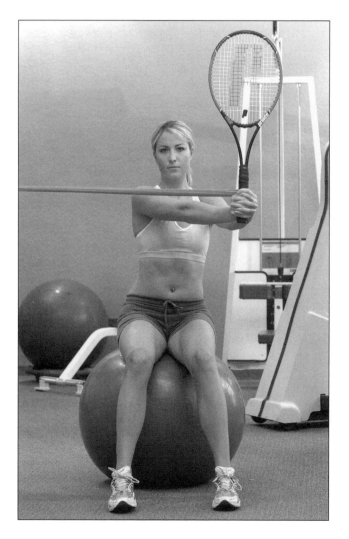

HORIZONTAL ABDUCTION (BACKHAND)
(Posterior Deltoid, Rotator Cuff, Scapular Muscles)

Secure or hold tubing at shoulder level. Grab other end with arm to be exercised. Place arms in position simulating a "high" one-handed backhand. Move racket arm forward and outward against resistance of band, keeping the other arm stationary. Slowly return.

Training Tip

Keep elbow firm and nearly straight to increase amount of work by shoulder.

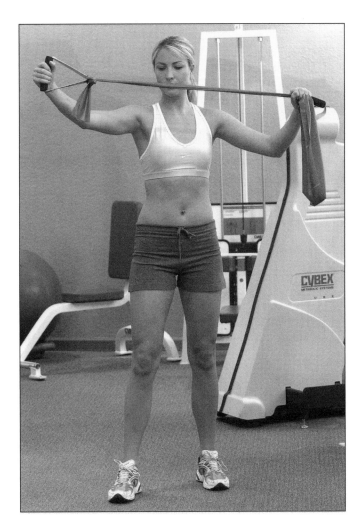

Golf

In golf, the most common injuries involve the wrist, hand, and lower back. The repetitive motions in these regions require stabilization from the muscles that cross these joints. Elastic resistance can be used to simulate the golf swing and provide sport specific resistance exercise options. The trunk and lower-extremity musculature accelerate the arms and club prior to impact, and share a key role in decelerating and stabilizing the body immediately after impact and during follow-through.

BASE EXERCISES

Shoulder internal and external rotation (page 20)

Diagonal extension (page 24)

Wrist flexion and extension (page 30)

Supination and pronation (page 32)

Trunk twist (page 62)

Hip internal and external rotation (page 88)

Squat (page 96)

SPORT SIMULATION EXERCISES

Golf-swing acceleration (page 180)

Golf-swing take-back with resistance (page 181)

GOLF-SWING ACCELERATION
(All Muscle Groups)

Assume golf stance. Secure band to stationary object at shoulder level. From take-back position, accelerate hands against band resistance to contact position. Slowly return.

Training Tip

Use lighter resistance levels to avoid compensating in patterns that aren't natural to golf swing.

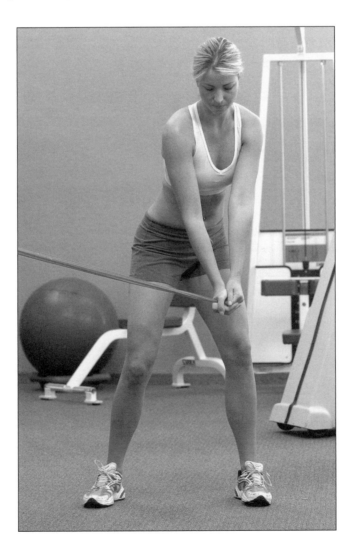

GOLF-SWING TAKE-BACK WITH RESISTANCE
(All Muscle Groups)

Secure long band or tubing under both feet. Grasp other end in both hands. In start position of swing and against resistance of band, move arms to take-back position of swing.

Training Tip

Use lighter resistance levels to avoid compensating in patterns that aren't natural to golf swing.

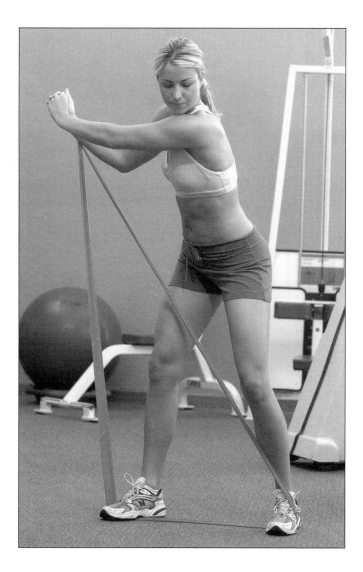

Skiing

Exceptional balance as well as muscular strength and endurance are required in the lower body of the skier. Despite advances in both ski and binding technology, knee injuries and fall-related trauma such as fractures and dislocations can occur. Skiers utilize sequences of lower-extremity muscle-action patterns to stabilize their joints and allow for turning and other agile maneuvers. High levels of muscle activity in the gluteals, quadriceps, and hamstrings, as well as the groin (adductors) and calf muscles, allow skiers to stabilize these joints, while maintaining proper control of their center of gravity over their oftentimes limited base of support. Programs to improve muscle strength and endurance have been widely recommended by top coaches and physicians who work not only with the world's top skiers, but also novices.

BASE EXERCISES

Hip flexion (page 82)

Hip extension (page 84)

Hip abduction (page 86)

Lunge (page 98)

Single-leg knee bend (page 183)

Balance squat with chair (page 184)

SPORT SIMULATION EXERCISES

Tuck squat (page 185)

Side to side lateral agility (page 186)

Double-leg resisted squat (page 187)

SINGLE-LEG KNEE BEND
(Gluteals, Quadriceps)

Stand on one leg with band or tubing secured under foot. Grasp other end of band and hold at waist level. Perform a one-leg squat bending knee 45 to 60 degrees. Slowly return.

Training Tips

Bend knee straight ahead and align knee cap with the second toe. Don't twist knee inward or outward. Maintain tension on band.

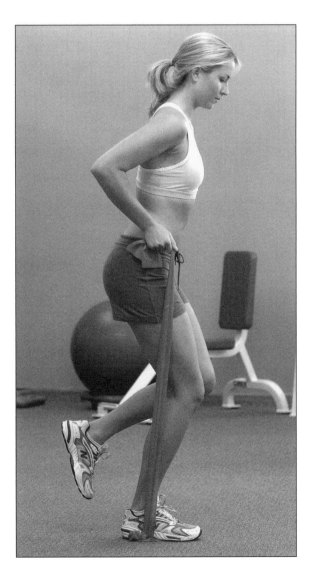

BALANCE SQUAT WITH CHAIR
(Gluteals, Quadriceps)

Stand on one leg with band or tubing secured under foot. Grasp other end of band and pull to waist level. Rest other leg on chair behind. Perform single leg squat, bending knee 45 to 60 degrees.

Training Tips

Remain upright and look straight ahead to optimally challenge balance systems of body. Maintain tension on band.

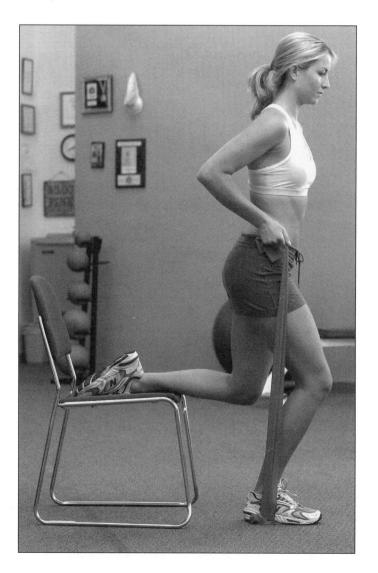

TUCK SQUAT (Core, Gluteals, Quadriceps)

Assume a "tuck" position with middle of long band wrapped around lower back. Secure bands under both feet to provide added resistance to the squat. Maintain tuck position while performing a mini-squat. Repeat.

Training Tip

A very small motion is used during squat because knees are already bent at starting position.

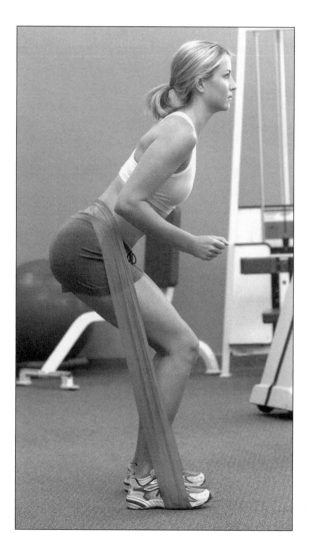

SIDE TO SIDE LATERAL AGILITY
(All Leg Muscles)

Secure one end of band at waist level on stationary object or with partner. Wrap band around waist and bound away from attachment point. Land on one leg, and briefly control that position. Slowly return.

Training Tip

Switch directions, and increase balance component by keeping the chin and head looking forward.

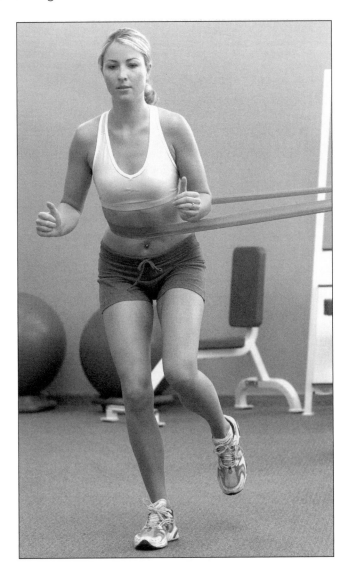

DOUBLE-LEG RESISTED SQUAT
(Quadriceps, Gluteals)

Stand on both legs with band secured under both feet. Grasp ends of band in both hands and wrap the band up over the top of the shoulders as pictured. Perform a partial squat looking straight ahead and minimizing any forward trunk bend. Slowly return to starting position and repeat.

Training Tips

Maintain proper trunk and hip alignment during the squat by looking straight ahead. Also, be sure that the knees remain properly aligned so that your kneecaps align over the middle of your toes as you descend.

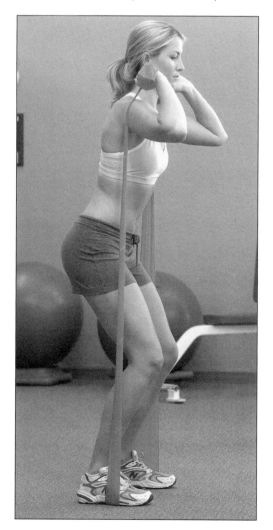

Swimming

The extremely repetitive nature of swimming can produce an exceptionally high number of overuse shoulder injuries. While swimmers compete in four primary strokes, the majority of a swimmer's training consists of the freestyle stroke. Repetitive stresses on the rotator cuff from both muscular fatigue as well as the overhead position of the shoulder make this area particularly vulnerable to injury. Exercises to strengthen the muscles responsible for the pull-through phase of swimming help to enhance performance, while exercises focusing on the rotator cuff and upper-back muscles help to promote muscular balance and prevent injury. High levels of muscular activity are needed in the muscles that flex and extend the hip and knee joint for kicking.

BASE EXERCISES

Shoulder internal and external rotation (page 20)

Seated row (page 38)

Shrug (page 46)

Hip flexion (page 82)

Hip extension (knee straight) (page 84)

Biceps curl at 90 degrees shoulder flexion (page 189)

SPORT SIMULATION EXERCISES

Pull-through (page 190)

Triceps extension (page 191)

BICEPS CURL AT 90 DEGREES SHOULDER FLEXION (Biceps)

Stand with shoulder flexed 90 degrees and band or tubing held in hand with other end secured to a door at shoulder height. Use the opposite arm placed under the elbow to support and stabilize the exercise motion. Begin with the elbow straight, and bend elbow against the resistance of the band or tubing to nearly end range. Slowly return to the starting position.

Training Tip

Because many athletes cannot fully straighten their elbow, don't force the elbow or bounce the elbow as it approaches full extension. Slowly control this part of the motion for safety and to get a greater benefit from the exercise.

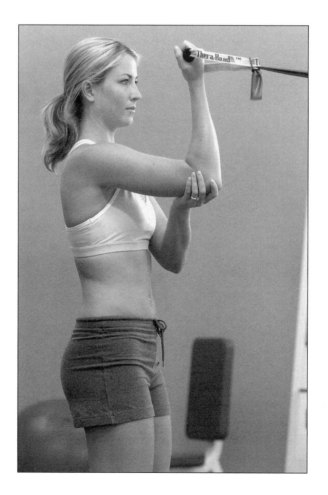

PULL-THROUGH (Latissimus Dorsi, Triceps)

Start with knees slightly bent and trunk bent forward to 90 degrees. Grab band or tubing in each hand with arms slightly forward and head in neutral position. Pull arms back, simulating pull-through phase of swimming and slowly return to starting position.

Training Tips

Squeeze shoulder blades together to increase activity of the shoulder blade muscles. Keep elbows straight and back in neutral alignment.

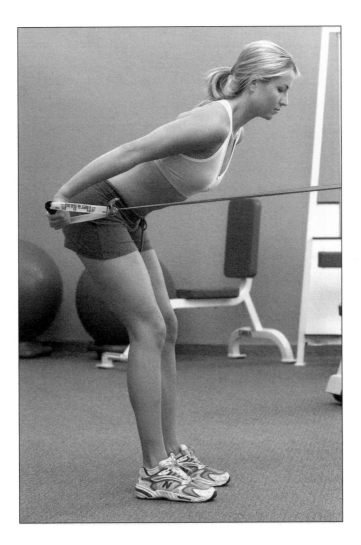

TRICEPS EXTENSION (SWIM POSITION)
(Triceps)

Grasp band or tubing with arms against sides and elbows bent 90 degrees. Bend forward at trunk with knees slightly bent. Extend arms until nearly straight. Slowly return.

Training Tips

Keep head and lower back in neutral alignment. Keep elbows by your side.

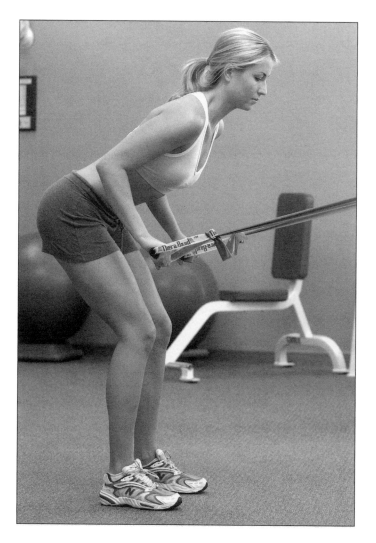

Running

Similar to swimming and other endurance sports, running requires exceptional muscular endurance to prevent overuse injuries. Additionally, running requires a stable pelvis and spine, so supplemental exercises are recommended for runners to improve core stability and hip strength. Since most running is truly "straight ahead," runners often benefit from side-to-side exercises to increase strength and stability of the hip, and also from exercises for the lower back and abdominals. Improving quadriceps and hamstring strength and endurance using a reasonably low-resistance level and high-repetition base is also recommended. Ankle strengthening exercises are also recommended to prevent ankle sprains that may occur during running. Finally, use of elastic resistance exercises for the upper-back and scapular muscles can benefit the long-distance runner as poor posture, fatigue, and discomfort in these areas can occur during training and ultra-long-distance events.

BASE EXERCISES

Seated row (page 38)

Shrug (page 46)

Curl-up (page 58)

Back extension (page 64)

Hip extension (page 84)

Squat (page 96)

Dorsiflexion (page 102)

Plantar flexion (page 104)

Ankle inversion (page 106)

Ankle eversion (page 108)

Hip abduction (page 186)

Side to side lateral agility (page 186)

Hockey

The combination of explosive power, balance, and agility can characterize the demands imposed on the athlete while playing hockey. Coupled with a unique training surface that is slippery, hockey places unique demands on the human musculoskeletal system. The nature of the ice creates tremendous eccentric, or lengthening, muscle contractions during skating with a high number of injuries in the hip and thigh region. Research has identified an optimal balance between the muscles that abduct and adduct the hip (outside hip muscles and groin muscles, respectively), with supplemental exercises recommended to better balance these important muscle groups. Finally, elastic resistance can help simulate sport-specific movements in both skating and shooting.

BASE EXERCISES

Monster walk (page 159)

Squat walk (page 194)

SPORT SIMULATION EXERCISES

Skating stride (page 195)

Resisted slide and stride (page 196)

Resisted slap shot take-back (page 197)

Resisted slap shot follow-through (page 198)

Wrist shot (page 199)

SQUAT WALK (All Muscle Groups)

Similar to monster walk (page 159). Loop band or tubing around lower leg or use an extremity strap to secure tubing to both ankles (pictured). With diagonal walking pattern, maintain flexed position of trunk and lower body.

Training Tip
Keep head up to avoid too much trunk bend. Maintain athletic posture.

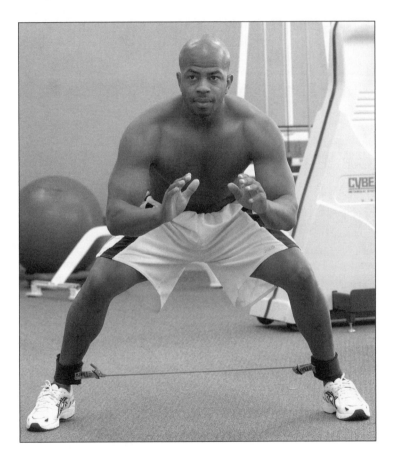

SKATING STRIDE (All Leg Muscles)

Loop band or tubing around lower leg or use an extremity strap to secure tubing to both ankles (pictured). Stride forward and diagonally, simulating the stride used during skating. Alternate limbs to most closely simulate the skating pattern.

Training Tips

Keep head looking forward to ensure that trunk does not bend too much. Perform exercise on a slide board to enhance movement.

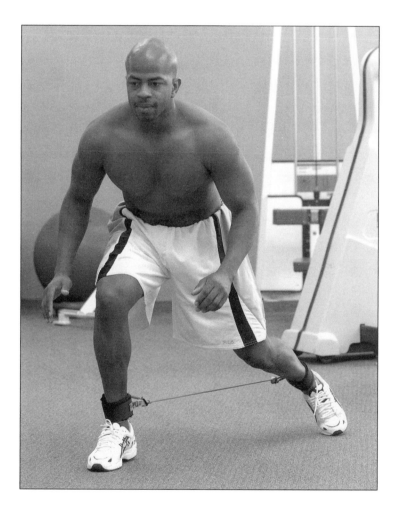

RESISTED SLIDE AND STRIDE
(Hip Abductors, Hip Adductors)

Stand beside a slide board or on tile floor. Loop band or tubing around lower leg or use an extremity strap to secure tubing to both ankles (pictured). Slide one leg to side while maintaining upright posture. Wear socks to facilitate sliding.

Training Tips

To increase the specificity of this exercise, hold hockey stick in both hands while performing. Keep back in neutral alignment and maintain athletic posture.

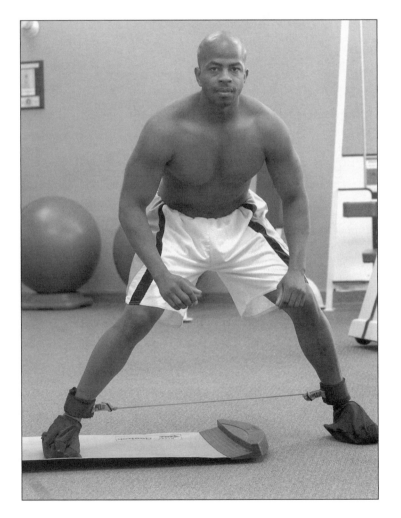

RESISTED SLAP SHOT (TAKE-BACK POSITION)
(All Muscle Groups)

Secure band or tubing around the end of hockey stick. Secure the other end so that take-back position of the slap shot is resisted as the stick is brought up away from the floor.

Training Tips

Avoid using too much resistance, which may produce an unnatural swing motion. Maintain neutral alignment of neck and back.

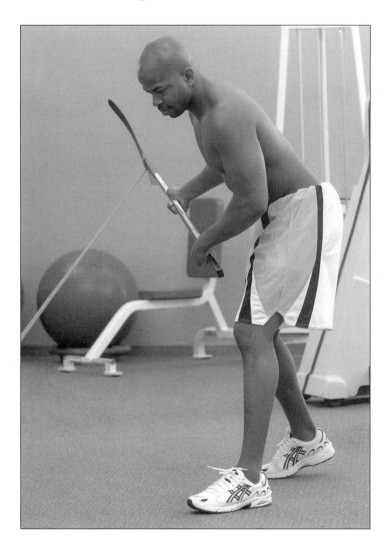

RESISTED SLAP SHOT (FOLLOW-THROUGH POSITION) (All Muscle Groups)

Secure band or tubing around end of hockey stick. Secure the other end so that band is 3 to 6 inches from floor. Move stick forward to simulate contact and end position of slap shot.

Training Tip

Altering location of tubing attachment to hockey stick will change resistance on wrists and forearms.

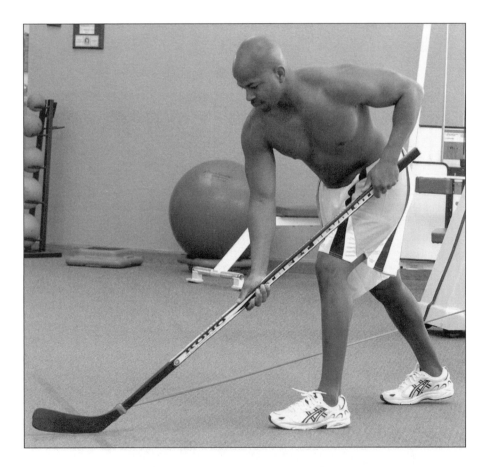

WRIST SHOT (START AND END POSITION)
(All Muscle Groups)

Secure tubing around end of hockey stick. Secure other end so that band is 3 to 6 inches from floor. Move the stick forward to simulate contact and end position of wrist shot.

Training Tip

Altering location of tubing attachment to hockey stick will change resistance on wrists and forearms.

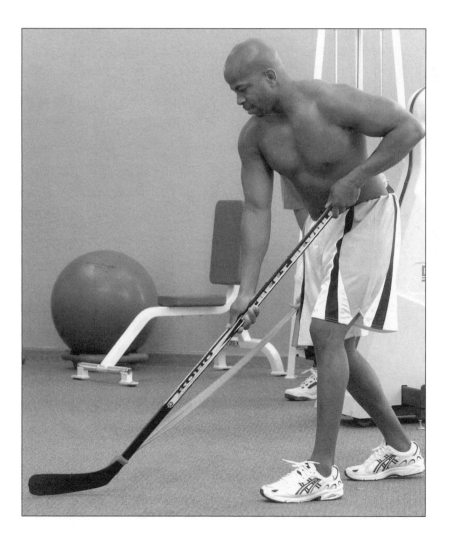

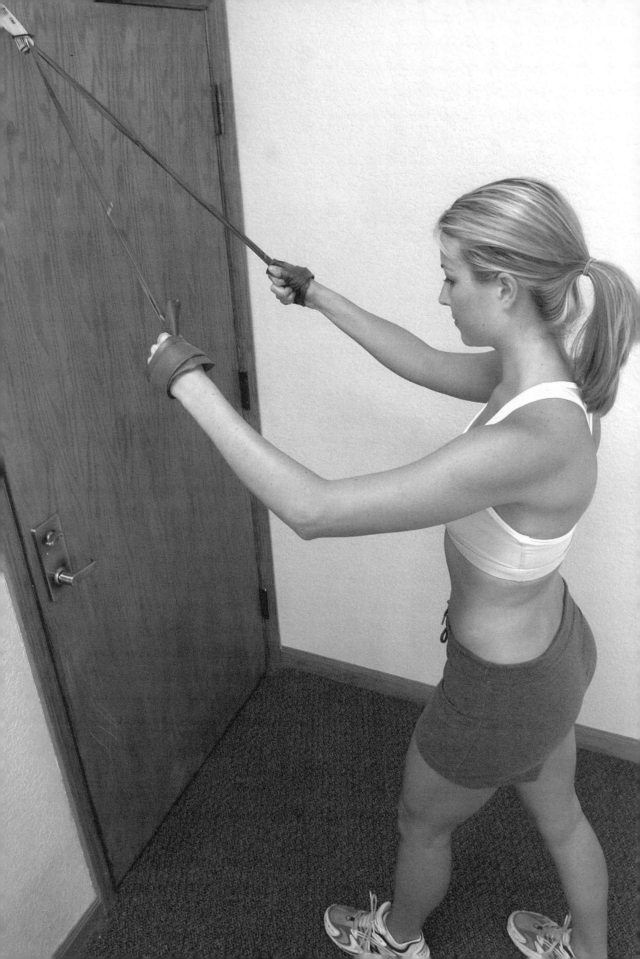

Chapter 11 . . . .

Training on the Road

One of the unique advantages of elastic resistance is its ability to provide a variable resistance to promote the development of muscular strength and endurance—and it is truly portable and compact. This makes elastic resistance training (ERT) optimal for travelers, because it allows them to take along a series of bands or tubing to most travel locations, whether a five-star hotel, athletic field, or tennis court.

Almost all of the exercises presented in this book can be used on the road in varying applications, and this chapter will demonstrate a very time-efficient program that can be done anywhere and with no ancillary equipment. Although many elastic resistance exercises can create a greater amount of simultaneous muscular activation (co-contraction) when performed on an exercise ball or while standing on a foam pad or unstable surface, carrying these exercise accessories is not a practical option for travelers. The exercises contained in this chapter are meant to utilize only the most portable elastic resistance equipment (bands and tubing) and can prove very useful for the average person or the athlete who travels. The sample travel exercises, in particular, are a way to continue balance and core training while on the road without the need for exercise machines. Using hotel objects such as pillows or towels for balance training to increase the difficulty of single-leg squats or other lower-body exercises is easily accomplished. Take care when anchoring the elastic material to hotel-room furniture because it may not be as strong or durable as the trusted bed frame or heavy desk at home.

While traveling, there's less time for training, so one important consideration in the traveling program is to include exercises that work multiple body segments and muscle groups at the same time. The term commonly used to describe this type of exercise is a multiple-joint exercise, as opposed to a single-joint exercise. This travel program contains several multiple-joint exercises that can optimize time and provide a more complete workout in a time-efficient manner. Multiple-joint exercises are typically functional and are recommended for both rehabilitation and performance training.

Another important consideration is to select exercises that work an area of emphasis. Because time constraints during travel may not allow a complete workout, it's important to prioritize an exercise program. One common example is to include exercises that work the quadriceps for a person with a history of knee problems. Using the same rationale, rotator cuff exercises for a tennis player or baseball player would be an essential ingredient in the traveling program. A sample generic program is listed in figure 11.1.

• •

Sample Travel Program Order

Upper Body

Bench press (page 36)

Lat pulldown (page 44)

Seated row (page 38)

Shoulder internal and external rotation (page 20)

Trunk

Abdominal crunch (performed with arms in 90/90 position with tubing anchored around desk leg or bedpost) (page 60)

Back extension (page 64)

Curl-up (page 58)

Trunk twist (page 62)

Lower body

Squat (page 96)

Single-leg knee bend (page 183)

Leg press (on couch) (page 94)

Knee flexion (page 92)

Plantar flexion (page 104)

Lateral step (page 156)

Side to side lateral agility (page 186)

Figure 11.1   Sample travel program.

Integrating the exercises in figure 11.1 with others in the book, based on time and the amount of space and resources in the travel environment, is highly recommended.

Finally, there may not be enough room to perform all of the most functional exercises in this book, so the exercises in this chapter are specifically designed to be performed in a limited space such as a hotel room, and they utilize simple anchor techniques for the elastic resistance material. Several products are available that allow the elastic material to be firmly attached to a doorjamb (see chapter 1) and will eliminate accidental slippage off a flimsy door handle or weak furniture. Safety is a key element in using elastic resistance exercises. When traveling, a bit of extra attention should be paid to ensuring that the door anchors or other methods of attaching are both adequate and effective.

Bibliography..........................

American College of Sports Medicine. 2000. *Guidelines for Exercise Testing and Prescription*. 6th edition. Lippincott Williams & Wilkins: Philadelphia.

Fleck, S.J., and Kraemer, W.J. 1997. *Designing Resistance Training Programs*. 2nd edition. Human Kinetics: Champaign, IL.

Geiger, U., and Schmid, C. 1998. *Muskeltraining mit dem Thera-Band*. BLV Verlagsgesellschaft mbH: Munich.

Kempf, H.D. 2000. *Rückentraining mit dem Thera-Band*. Reinbek: Hamburg.

Kempf, H.D., and Lowis, A. 1999. *Fit und Schön mit dem Thera-Band*. Reinbek: Hamburg.

Kempf, H.D., Schmelcher, F., and Ziegler, C. 1996. *Trainingsbuch Thera-Band*. Reinbek: Hamburg.

Kempf, H.D., and Strack, A. 1999. *Krafttraining mit dem Thera-Band*. Reinbek: Hamburg.

Page, P., and Ellenbecker, T. (eds.). 2003. *The Scientific and Clinical Application of Elastic Resistance*. Human Kinetics: Champaign, IL.

Page, et al. 2000. Clinical force production of Thera-Band elastic bands. *J Orthop Sports Phys Ther*. (abstract) 30(1):A47–8.

Wnuck, A. 1999. *Bodytrainer Tubing*. Reinbek: Hamburg.

About the Authors...................

Phil Page, MS, PT, ATC, CSCS, is a physical therapist, athletic trainer, and certified strength and conditioning specialist. He is the manager of clinical education and research for Thera-Band Products and has a private practice in Baton Rouge, Louisiana, specializing in sports and orthopedic physical therapy.

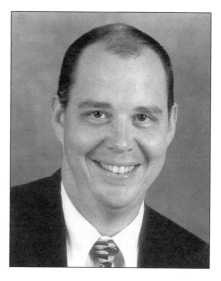

Page has worked with the NFL's New Orleans Saints and Seattle Seahawks and the athletic programs at Tulane University. He has lectured internationally on the scientific and clinical use of elastic resistance and developed an educational course on elastic resistance that is being taught in six countries.

He is certified by the National Athletic Trainers' Association (NATA) and was awarded the NATA's Otto Davis Postgraduate Scholarship in 1991. He is coauthor of *The Scientific and Clinical Application of Elastic Resistance* (Human Kinetics, 2003).

Page lives in Baton Rouge, Louisiana, with his wife and three children.

Todd Ellenbecker, MS, PT, SCS, OCS, CSCS, is the clinic director at Physiotherapy Associates Scottsdale Sports Clinic in Scottsdale, Arizona. A licensed physical therapist, he has researched and taught in the field for 18 years.

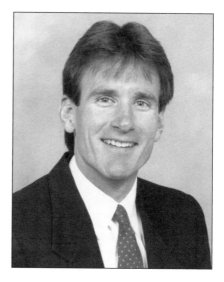

Ellenbecker is certified by the American Physical Therapy Association (APTA) as both a sports clinical specialist and orthopedic clinical specialist. The APTA also awarded him its Sports Physical Therapy Clinical Teaching Award in 1999. He was chairman of the APTA's Shoulder Special Interest Group and is a manuscript reviewer for the *Journal of Orthopaedic and Sports Physical Therapy* and *American Journal of Sports Medicine.*

In addition, Ellenbecker is a member of the American College of Sports Medicine (ACSM) and the United States Professional Tennis Association (USPTA). He is chairman of the United States Tennis Association's (USTA) National Sport Science Committee and is a certified strength and conditioning specialist through the National Strength and Conditioning Association (NSCA). In 2003, the NSCA named him the Sports Medicine Professional of the Year.

He has served as a member of the Thera-Band research advisory committee and is coauthor of *The Scientific and Clinical Application of Elastic Resistance*. He also has cowritten *The Elbow in Sport*, *Complete Conditioning for Tennis*, and *Closed Kinetic Chain Exercise*.

Ellenbecker lives in Scottsdale, Arizona, with his wife, Gail.